Advance Praise for Dignity in Care

This wonderful book is the result of the lifelong clinical and academic journey of one of the giants in psycho-oncology and palliative care. The book is packed with practical and inspiring stories and recommendations. Everyone involved in healthcare must read this book to better help patients and families and to infuse more meaning and fulfillment into their own practice.

Eduardo Bruera, MDFT McGraw Chair in the Treatment of Cancer
Chair, Department of Palliative, Rehabilitation, & Integrative Medicine
UT MD Anderson Cancer Center

Dr. Chochinov has gathered his decades of clinical experience and wisdom and distilled it into this gift to the field of healthcare, *Dignity in Care: The Human Side of Medicine*. The book is rich in stories of patients and their families, and in the deep narratives of the clinicians who care for them. He has written eloquently about the pillars of patient-centered care, including the patient experience of illness, communication, and dignity-affirming care. The book speaks to all disciplines and is a tribute to Dr. Chochinov's very distinguished career and to his enduring contribution to advance our understanding of the concept of dignity and why it is so critical in these challenging times. It is vital reading for novices to experts.

Betty Ferrell, RN, PhD, FAAN, FPCN, CHPN
Professor, City of Hope Medical Center
PI, End of Life Nursing Education Consortium (ELNEC)

Dr. Chochinov has spent a long and highly distinguished career caring about people while he has been providing care to patients—most of whom have cancer. In *Dignity in Care: The Human Side of Medicine*, Dr. Chochinov helps us understand why and how dignified caring for persons has to be a part of effective healthcare. In story after story, he shows us the consequences of not providing this care and what healing can happen when true caring does happen. This is a book that both inspires and gives us practical tools to provide dignity in care. It is a must-read for every healthcare provider.

The Rev. George Handzo, APBCC, CSSBB Director,
Health Services Research & Quality HealthCare Chaplaincy Network

Bolstered by decades of research and richly illustrated with vignettes of people's lived experiences, *Dignity in Care: The Human Side of Medicine* illuminates the tenets of authentic human caring. Dr. Chochinov reminds us that, even in the midst of suffering, feeling out of control and utterly vulnerable, the inherent dignity of each patient is there—if we take the time and hone the skill to recognize it. This book is such an important contribution to the field of medicine.

Ira Byock, MD, Active Emeritus Professor, Dartmouth Geisel School of Medicine,
author of *Dying Well* and *the Best Care Possible*

Dr. Chochinov is a global leader in palliative care and a tireless advocate for honoring the dignity of all patients entrusted to our care. Patients with chronic and serious illness can become trapped in their physical illness story within healthcare systems which afford no room for the inner story of the patient to be heard—the story of meaning, purpose, strength, and deep worth—the essence of being more than one's illness. *Dignity in Care: The Human Side of Medicine*, provides the tools and resources for all clinicians and caregivers to elicit and be present to the powerful stories of patients, which often go unheard, and in so doing ensure that the dignity of all patients is honored throughout their care. This book is an important gift to everyone training or working in healthcare.

Christina Puchalski, MD, MS, FACP, FAAHPM
Professor of Medicine and Health Sciences
Exec Director, George Washington University Institute for Spirituality and Health
George Washington University
Washington, DC

In *Dignity in Care: The Human Side of Medicine*, Dr. Harvey Max Chochinov offers insight into a critical piece of healthcare: how to recognize, respect, and affirm the humanity of patients and their families. Drawing on decades of personal experience in psychosocial oncology, Dr. Chochinov elucidates the complexity of the physician–patient relationship. He encourages healthcare providers to adopt a holistic approach to understand how patients and families experience profound changes in their health. A sensitive and empathic exploration of an overlooked topic, *Dignity in Care* presents a particularly important perspective as we continue to battle the COVID-19 pandemic.

L. Trevor Young, MD, PhD, FRCPC, FCAHS
Dean and Vice Provost, Temerty Faculty of Medicine
University of Toronto

Dignity in Care: The Human Side of Medicine is an essential therapeutic treasure map for any healthcare professional committed to preserving and expanding what it means to be a person in the context of serious illness. Gifted clinician, teacher, and researcher Harvey Max Chochinov, MD, psychiatrist, and supportive care pioneer, creatively integrates actual case studies with clinical instruments and models. He blends multiple healing stories that, at their very core, are as relevant for patients and families as they are for healthcare professionals. This book is a serious look at the heart and soul of what it means to be human and specific ways to deeply connect with people in distress through emotional connection, dignity, trust, and agency. Boldly, Dr. Chochinov also unveils the barriers and opportunities in healthcare education and hospitals to humanize the illness experience. *Dignity in Care: The Human Side of Medicine* is first and foremost about clinical care. Dr. Chochinov deftly distills and shares the best compilation of how to provide dignity in care to date. The added bonus is the robust psychological, social, and spiritual growth implications for all of us.

Matthew Loscalzo, LCSW, APOS Fellow
Executive Director, People & Enterprise Transformation
Emeritus Professor Supportive Care Medicine
Professor Population Sciences
City of Hope-National Medical Center

Reading Dr. Chochinov's *Dignity in Care: The Human Side of Medicine* is like experiencing a master clinician's class in how to establish and nourish the clinician–patient relationship to assure dignity in care. This innovative text, written by an eminent psychiatrist and researcher, should be essential reading for all healthcare professionals as they embark on their clinical encounters. The readable format with clinical anecdotes, personal reflections, research data, and memorable ABCD core competencies provides profound and practical insights into the concepts of personhood and patienthood. The book emphasizes the need for healthcare professionals to understand the patient's illness context and the complexities and variables that influence their vulnerability and impact their sense of dignity. But it does much more than define these concepts. It offers an evidenced-based therapeutic communication framework to address the range of aspects of dignity-related stress. There is a brilliance and simplicity to creating an environment for delivering dignity in care, and this text uniquely advances a way forward for healthcare professionals to intentionally integrate this approach into their patient encounters and expand their therapeutic armamentarium. This book will have a profound influence on how we strive to achieve dignity in care for all.

Kathleen M. Foley, MD

Member Emeritus, Memorial Sloan Kettering Cancer Center

Professor Emeritus, Department of NeurologyWeill Cornell Medical School

Dignity in Care

The Human Side of Medicine

Harvey Max Chochinov

Distinguished Professor of Psychiatry, University of Manitoba

Senior Scientist, CancerCare Manitoba Research Institute

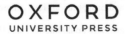

OXFORD
UNIVERSITY PRESS

OXFORD
UNIVERSITY PRESS

Library of Congress Cataloging-in-Publication Data
Names: Chochinov, Harvey Max, author.
Title: Dignity in care : the human side of medicine / Harvey Max Chochinov.
Description: New York, NY : Oxford University Press, 2023. |
Includes bibliographical references and index.
Identifiers: LCCN 2022020993 (print) | LCCN 2022020994 (ebook) |
ISBN 9780199380428 (hardback) | ISBN 9780197798133 (paperback) |
ISBN 9780199380442 (epub) | ISBN 9780199380459
Subjects: MESH: Patient Care Management—ethics | Patients—psychology |
Physician-Patient Relations | Personhood | Respect | Patient-Centered Care
Classification: LCC RA971 (print) | LCC RA971 (ebook) | NLM W 84.7 |
DDC 362.1068—dc23/eng/20220819
LC record available at https://lccn.loc.gov/2022020993
LC ebook record available at https://lccn.loc.gov/2022020994

DOI: 10.1093/med/9780199380428.001.0001

Paperback printed by Integrated Books International, United States of America

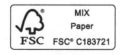

To my wife Michelle and our remarkable children, Lauren, Rachel, and our soon to be son-in-law, Cam.
In memory of my dear mother Shirley Chochinov, sister Ellen Chochinov and Joyce Basman—never to be forgotten.

Contents

Preface for Paperback Edition

Rarely do I deliver a lecture or a workshop where the question of dignity and cross-cultural resonance is not raised. People want to know if the notion of dignity in care is culturally bound; that is, whether these ideas apply to certain groups of people and perhaps less well to others. Extensive research of dignity-informed practices over the last few decades offers a fascinating and informed response. While cultural nuances, adaptations, and translations have been an important part of this work, what is most telling, and moving, is how the basic ideas underpinning dignity in care have taken hold worldwide: ideas like feeling acknowledged as whole persons; feeling valued and respected; being able to tap into aspects of ourselves that make us feel worthwhile and complete; being able to safeguard the well-being of those we love and care about most; being aware of our own vulnerability and mortality; and hoping our lives will make a difference in a world we must all eventually leave behind. Those are not culturally specific ideas or constructs, but rather universal threads sewn into the fabric of our collective humanity and the essence of what it means to be human.

When we are ill, or threatened by loss of health, those core elements of self—our essence if you will—take on heightened importance, meaning, and poignancy. As physical or emotional vitality wanes, people strive to safeguard facets of themselves that illness cannot touch. While the entirety of medicine is organized around determining why someone gets sick and what might be done to restore well-being, dignity in care insists on never losing sight of the person, despite whatever limitations or incumbrances their ailment imposes. "I am not my illness"; "I am not my tumor"; "I am not my disability." Finding ways to affirm whole persons, and not allowing patienthood to eclipse personhood, is what *Dignity in Care: The Human Side of Medicine* is all about.

Since this book came out, there have been some interesting publications further informing how to understand and practice dignity in care. The article "Intensive Caring: Reminding Patients They Matter"[1] was inspired by the words of Dame Cicely Saunders, the founder of the modern hospice movement, who famously said, "You matter because you are you, and you matter to the last moment of your life." While this has become the central philosophical tenet of palliative care, it doesn't describe how to offer care that reminds patients they matter. *Intensive Caring* was designed to fill that gap and cites many of the empirical approaches described in *Dignity in Care: The Human Side of Medicine*. Just as intensive care describes a response to patients in dire physical distress, *Intensive Caring* offers ways to address patients in dire emotional, existential, or spiritual distress, who may be feeling hopeless, helpless, and that their lives no longer matter. The elements described in *Intensive Caring* include nonabandonment, taking an interest in the patient as a person, holding or containing hope for patients when they can no longer do so for themselves, providing a dignity-conserving tone of care (as is described in this book in the chapter on optimal therapeutic effectiveness), and therapeutic humility. *Intensive Caring* challenges the conventional medical paradigm—*examine, diagnose, and fix*—acknowledging that many facets of human suffering cannot be fixed. Hence, it sees *examine* yield to finding out who patients are as persons; *diagnosis* yield to understanding the nature of their suffering; and *fix* yield to offering comfort and trusting the therapeutic process in the service of healing. These are entirely consistent with the core principles and components of dignity in care.

Another recently published paper[2] introduces the concept of *fractured personhood*, referring to a shattered sense of core self and identity, wherein life becomes unsustainable. In other words, wanting to die emerges within a state of brokenness marked by dissatisfaction, contempt, and rejection of who we are, relative to who we were or want to be. This might occur by way of illness, calamity, or trauma, with feeling intact, autonomy, and resilience yielding to a sense of inadequacy, self-loathing, and a compulsion to self-destruct. Fractured personhood could help us understand suicidality and speaks to the importance of safeguarding *integrity of personhood*, detailed in the chapter "The ABCDs of Dignity Conserving Care."

Another paper[3] published after *Dignity in Care* warns against the pitfalls of black and white thinking, emphasizing the importance of myriad issues affecting human suffering, including the white, the black, and all shades in between. This book delves into the complexities and nuances of providing dignity in care. While it includes models, algorithms, and frameworks informing this approach, it is not reductionistic, recognizing the uniqueness of each person. If one hard-and-fast rule applies across dignity in care, it is the title of a paper I published a decade ago entitled " The Secret Is Out: Patients Are People with Feelings That Matter."[4] Too often, healthcare is reduced to a set of core activities, responsibilities, and tasks, which over time can become robotic, mechanistic, and removed from the human connectedness that makes the difference between healthcare and *healthcaring*.

Recently, a group of colleagues from around the world published an article entitled "Top Ten Tips Palliative Care Clinicians Should Know About Dignity-Conserving Practice."[5] In a concise and clear fashion, this paper summarizes much of the work I have done over three decades related to dignity. The tips read as follows:

Tip 1: Dignity is affirmed through specific and consistent clinician behaviors that can be taught and learned and adapted to the clinician's practice.

Tip 2: Dignity is preserved, promoted, and protected, in part, by the nature of the overall care setting.

Tip 3: Every person experiences dignity and indignity differently—it is the clinician's responsibility to find out what dignity means to each person, here and now.

Tip 4: Dignity-conserving care can relieve suffering by addressing loneliness, desire for hastened death, and existential distress, among other challenges.

Tip 5: Dignity-based palliative care affirms patients' unique qualities and worth, thus supporting self-actualization, autonomy, and critical values.

Tip 6: Several simple, brief, and useful tools to support the person's sense of dignity have been developed and show beneficial effects.

Tip 7: Dignity therapy has a positive impact on the emotional and social well-being of patients and those receiving legacy documents.

Tip 8: The Patient Dignity Question can serve as a core palliative care practice to anchor the relationship with patients in what is most important to them as human beings.

Tip 9: Dignity-conserving care takes many forms throughout a disease course and must be adapted to the person, population, culture, and context.

Tip 10: Dignity-conserving practice can help dismantle palliative care clinicians' biases, thus enhancing the tone of care and maintaining a person-centered lens.

These ten tips collectively describe the essence of dignity in care. Like this book, I hope they can be applied in the service of moving the culture of medicine toward a kinder, more compassionate, person-centered approach.

Since this book was published, the world has witnessed too much hatred, too much pain, too much sorrow. As is often the case, these destructive forces take hold and obliterate our ability to appreciate and honor all we hold in common, allowing differences to set us asunder. Within our work, we have an opportunity to transcend base instincts, and value people, regardless of race, creed, or color, for who they are as whole persons. While it is easy to yield to cynicism and despair, by treating our patients and each other with kindness and respect, individually and collectively, in our own small way, we bend the arc of the universe toward hope, healing, and peace.

Harvey Max Chochinov
December 18, 2024
Winnipeg, Canada

References

1. Chochinov HM. Intensive caring: Reminding patients they matter. J Clin Oncol. 2023; 41:2884–2887.
2. Chochinov HM. *Fractured Personhood*, Suicide, and lessons from those nearing death. J Palliat Med. 2023 Aug; 26(8):1037–1039.
3. Chochinov HM. Response to Downar J et al., Medical assistance in dying and palliative care: Shared trajectories. J Palliat Med. 2023; 26:1319.
4. Chochinov HM. The secret is out: Patients are people with feelings that matter. Palliat Support Care. 2013; 11:287–288.
5. Hadler RA, Weeks S, Rosa WE, Choate S, Goldshore M, Julião M, Mergler B, Nelson J, Soodalter J, Zhuang C, Chochinov HM. Top ten tips palliative care clinicians should know about dignity-conserving practice. J Palliat Med. 2023 Oct; 27(4):537–544.

Preface

For many reasons, 1986 was a particularly memorable year. On a personal front, it marked the birth of my daughter Lauren Jessie. Along with her younger sister Rachel Erin, born 4 years later, fatherhood was and remains a profound, life-changing blessing, second to none. This was also the year I moved to New York City to begin my training in psycho-oncology, a discipline devoted to understanding the psychological dimensions of cancer, at Memorial Sloan Kettering Cancer Center. Up until then, most of my education had been in Winnipeg, Canada. There I completed my medical degree, followed by a residency in the Department of Psychiatry at the University of Manitoba. Somewhere along the way, it struck me that the psychological care of patients with cancer was largely being ignored and that their needs were enormous. After exploring where I might learn more about this, all fingers pointed toward Sloan Kettering and the Department of Psychiatry led by Dr. Jimmie Holland. Dr. Holland was a preeminent, global pioneer and founder in the field of psycho-oncology.

Training at Memorial Sloan Kettering meant being mentored by the likes of Jimmie Holland, William Breitbart, Kathleen Foley, Jerome Posner, and Nessa Coyle, each one a leader and innovator whose inspiration has shaped more than three decades of my professional life. In 1986, I knew very little about looking after patients with cancer and had virtually no experience in palliative care. Becoming a fellow in psycho-oncology, with a primary assignment to the neuro-oncology ward, changed all of that. I began caring for patients with life-threatening and life-limiting cancers and started hearing their stories and observing their particular ways of coping. For some, the diagnosis of cancer was the beginning of a spiritual journey marked by acceptance, magnanimity, and personal growth. For others it heralded the untethering of a sense of self, sometimes undermining their will to live in the face of uncertainty and declining health. This was also the height of the AIDS crisis, with New York being at the epicenter. Those of us working in psychiatry struggled to support patients and families navigating this mysterious illness, along with helping them face a tsunami of loss and grief.

Upon completing my fellowship, I returned to Winnipeg to help launch a Department of Psychosocial Oncology at CancerCare Manitoba, which has provided emotional support services to patients with cancer and their families for nearly 35 years. With the encouragement and collaboration of a profoundly capable mentor, Dr. Keith Wilson, I also launched a program of research exploring the vast experiential landscape of palliative and end-of-life care for patients and their families. I am forever grateful to all my collaborators affiliated with the Manitoba Palliative Care Research Unit. Collectively we authored several hundred publications, investigating diverse topics such as depression, desire for death, will to live, hopelessness, sense of burden, personhood, communication, and a whole program of research focused on patient dignity. I have also been privileged to co-edit the *Handbook of Psychiatry in Palliative Medicine* (Oxford University Press) with my dear friend and *brother*, William Breitbart. The third edition of this seminal text is currently being prepared and should be published next year. I like to think it has galvanized the field of palliative psychiatry and helped inform and guide a new generation of clinicians and researchers interested in the emotional dimensions of palliative care.

Over the past 35 years I have learned a few things about looking after patients and what it means to provide *Dignity in Care*. As I enter the twilight of my career, this seemed like the right time to write this book about the human side of medicine and share insights acquired over decades, making them available to anyone whose work or experience brings them into close contact with patients and their families. While I have largely looked after patients with cancer and those in palliative care, the information, skills, and insights I hope to share implicates all patients, in all settings. If you are a doctor, nurse, social worker, hospital chaplain, occupational therapist, physiotherapist, physician's assistant, healthcare aide, x-ray technologist, radiation therapist, respiratory therapist, pharmacist, dentist, dental assistant or hygienist, medical receptionist, healthcare trainee of any kind—or a patient or family member interested in dignity in care—this book has been written for you.

I have organized the book into four chapters, each crafted to provide readers with the requisite knowledge and skills needed to achieve dignity in care. The first chapter, "Understanding Patienthood," sets the stage by offering readers an appreciation of what shapes patients' responses to changing health circumstances and their encounters with healthcare providers and healthcare systems. This is important, given that we need to know why someone is reacting as they are before drilling down into how to respond to them. The second chapter, "The ABCDs of Dignity-Conserving Care," acknowledges that everyone working in healthcare brings certain innate qualities, outlooks, and ways of engaging with patients that profoundly shape each clinical encounter. Attitude, behavior, compassion, and dialogue address core competencies we must be mindful of to achieve dignity in care. Chapter 3, "The

Model of Optimal Therapeutic Communication," provides a unique, data-driven model of effective communication, akin to an anatomical dissection of what makes clinical encounters work. This model brings together the need to understand patient responses (Chapter 1), while invoking healthcare provider approaches and characteristics (Chapter 2), leading to optimal therapeutic communication. It is based on the collective input and wisdom of scores of healthcare professionals and offers guidance and direction for achieving dignity in care. Finally, Chapter 4, "Dignity in Care," is a culmination of insights and approaches based on a program of research that engaged hundreds of patients exploring what supports or undermines their sense of dignity. The Model of Dignity and innovations such as the Patient Dignity Inventory and Dignity Therapy describe evidence-based approaches that can inform anyone in healthcare about how to be attentive to patient dignity, whatever their current healthcare challenges may be.

I have thought about these ideas for a very long time and spent years doing research that has shaped my thinking and clinical practice. Besides learning from my patients, I've also been influenced and inspired by many sage colleagues whose voices and stories I have recorded and shared within the pages of this book. I believe I now understand the intricacies and nuances of how to provide patients with respectful, affirming, kind, *Dignity in Care*. It's taken me a few decades to sort all of this out and put these pieces together. Hopefully reading this book will help you do so sooner.

About the Author

Harvey Max Chochinov is Distinguished Professor of Psychiatry at the University of Manitoba and a senior scientist at CancerCare Manitoba Research Institute. His research provides an empirical basis for understanding and addressing palliative and end-of-life care experiences for patients and their families. His more than 350 career publications have broached diverse topics such as communication, depression, quality-of-life, suicide, vulnerability, spirituality, and existential distress toward end of life. He also has led a large program of research targeting issues related to dignity within the healthcare setting. He is the co-founder of the Canadian Virtual Hospice, which is the world's largest repository of web-based information and support for dying patients, their families, and healthcare providers. He is the editor of *The Handbook of Psychiatry in Palliative Medicine* (Oxford University Press) and co-editor of the journal *Supportive and Palliative Care* (Cambridge University Press). His book, *Dignity Therapy: Final Words for Final Days*, was the 2011 winner of the Prose Award. He has received top research awards from the Canadian Psychiatric Association, the Canadian Cancer Society, the American Association of Hospice and Palliative Care, and the International Psycho-oncology Society; a lifetime achievement award from the Canadian Association of Psychosocial Oncology; and the highest honor that can be bestowed by the Canadian Medical Association, the FNG Starr Award. He is an Order of Manitoba recipient and an Officer in the Order of Canada. In 2020, he was inducted into the Canadian Medical Hall of Fame.

Introduction

A few years ago, the physician-in-chief of our hospital, Dr. Perry Gray, circulated a note of complaint from the wife of a patient who had been cared for in our facility. The note described how her husband had been brought to the emergency room by ambulance, admitted to hospital, and shortly thereafter died. She indicated that most of his care was satisfactory and, in some instances, even excellent—with one significant exception. Soon after arriving in hospital, his CT scan had shown that his lung cancer had spread to his abdomen, and he and the family were told to prepare themselves for the worst. Regular doses of morphine were started to alleviate his pain. He survived the night and early the next morning was still able to answer questions from his oncologist. Shortly thereafter, he slipped into unconsciousness.

> Sometime between 10:00 and 11:00 that morning, the medical students and residents were scheduled to do rounds. They met in the room situated directly across the hall from his room, then came out into the hallway and stood immediately outside his door. He was in Bed 2 beside the window. His parents and I were sitting beside him and the curtain was drawn between us and the patient in Bed 1. In the hallway, I heard someone say, "Bed 1 is Mrs. X and Bed 2 is Mr. -----." I was focused on my husband and did not hear what was said next about Mrs. X. I then clearly heard a male voice say "Mr. -----" and a second male voice say, "Well, I guess we could go in and see if he's still alive." Another male voice laughed and then the group moved down the hallway. I cannot tell you how painful this was to me. Despite his illness, my husband's death was sudden and unexpected. To hear him dismissed in such a callous manner was devastating. Perhaps a middle-aged man in a coma is not an "interesting" case, but Denis was a loving and much-beloved husband, son, brother, and uncle. He deserved far more respect than he was shown by these students. The initial comment, the laugh, and the lack of reprimand of any kind from the person in charge led me to question the care that he'd received, and that future patients will receive, from this group of future doctors.

As Physician-in-Chief, Dr. Gray is often in touch with the medical staff. He told me that no other correspondence had ever elicited the kind of response

he received after circulating this letter. Many colleagues approached him offering reassure that *it wasn't them.* Perhaps even more telling was that many
confessed that, while it wasn't them, *it very well could have been.*

No one goes into healthcare with the intention of hurting people or wanting
to come across as callous, cold, or unfeeling. Fortunately, most people
working in healthcare understand that kindness and compassion are key, even
foundational, to being successful in caring for patients and their families. And
yet, all too often, there are instances when contact with healthcare is tainted
by experiences ranging from vaguely annoying or abrasive to outright emotionally assaultive. Patients may encounter challenges that chip away at their
sense of self and pride. This can be as subtle as being kept waiting for an appointment; as insidious as having to wear a plastic hospital bracelet that tracks
patients according to an institutional number or code; as jarring as being referred to on the basis of a body part gone wrong, the proverbial "GI bleed in
Room 2" or "breast tumor in Room 3"; or as devastating as feeling that their
anguish or fear is not being recognized or somehow stopped being heard over
the unrelenting din of modern-day medicine.

Admittedly some issues are hard to avoid. Providing care to the masses
requires that certain sacrifices be made, often in the name of efficiency.
Patients' schedules must often accommodate professional availability.
Personal preferences, for those in institutional settings such as hospitals or
personal care homes—whether for mealtimes, bedtimes, or bath times—must
yield to some degree to organizational protocols and staffing considerations.
And while regulations, conformity, and standardization have their place
and are necessary to sustain viable healthcare systems, they can be tough on
patients in that they force them to relinquish a certain amount of control and
choice in exchange for getting the care they need. Little wonder that the word
"patience," to endure without complaint, and "patient" come from the same
Latin derivative *patientem,* referring to "a willingness to bear adversities, calm
endurance of misfortune and suffering." Clearly it takes great patience to be a
patient, and the sicker you are and the more care you need, the more your patience may be put to the test.

Being a patient can assault one's sense of self. When *who you are* matters less
or is perceived to matter less than the specifics of your ailment, patienthood
threatens to eclipse personhood. Anyone with patient contact is implicated
in this crucial dynamic, be they the physician who performs an examination
or does a procedure, the medical receptionist who answers the telephone
or books an appointment, the housekeeper who cleans the hospital room,
the triage nurse who determines an appropriate medical disposition, or the
healthcare aide who assists with intimacies of care such as bathing, dressing,

and toileting. While each has a specific role to play and various tasks to perform, any one of them can fundamentally rescue the way an interaction is experienced by making patients feel that they matter, that someone cares, and that no one is indifferent to their anguish or fear or vulnerability. I recall once walking into the room of a young woman with an aggressive leukemia, suffering from complications of a bone marrow transplant. The housekeeper, whom I had seen daily during my regular ward rounds, was standing at her bedside, quietly cleaning the room. She looked up when I walk in, tears in her eyes, to tell me "she's not doing so good today." It struck me that this housekeeper would never show indifference that might cause someone to feel like a piece of furniture, just another object to be swept, mopped, or dusted around.

Satisfaction with healthcare starts to unravel when the tasks of care trump attentiveness to the person being cared for. The explanations for why this happens and what can be done to prevent it are complicated. It is highly doubtful, for instance, that the medical staff involved in Denis's care are bad people; the fact that so many people told Dr. Gray that "it could have been them" suggests that something quite common happens in healthcare, causing people to tune out the human drama and pathos of working in close proximity to sickness, suffering, and death. Dr. Daniel D. Federman, Dean of Medical Education at Harvard Medical School, suggests that *there is something about medical education and something about what the students go through which blunts this empathy with which they arrive.*[1] And although this may be common, as far as patients are concerned, it exacts a considerable price. For patients it can mean feeling dismissed, misunderstood, or otherwise overlooked. For healthcare professionals, it can mean relinquishing the very motivation that attracted most of them into this work in the first place—the chance to connect with people and demonstrate their humanity and compassion within the field of healthcare.

For those tempted to read no further, here is the bottom line. *Patients are people with feelings that matter.*[2] Anyone who chooses to work in healthcare and is in contact with patients simply cannot afford to forget this. Patients are people. People have feelings. And those feelings matter. While it may sound simple, perhaps even trite, it is often underappreciated, easily overlooked, and tragically forgotten. That is what happened the morning Denis died. No one was trying to hurt his feelings or those of his wife and family. No one was knowingly trying to inflict further pain on these people facing the loss of a man they loved. These healthcare providers were likely just trying to make their way through another hectic day, preoccupied with getting through ward rounds, reviewing recent blood work, interpreting diagnostic tests, deliberating treatment decisions, organizing discharge plans—just a busy day, like almost every other day, on a typical medical ward. However, despite all this frenetic activity and attention being paid to countless details, the human tragedy that was unfolding in Bed 2 next to the window was simply not on their radar.

If you are training or working in healthcare in any capacity whatsoever and have contact with patients, *Dignity in Care: The Human Side of Medicine*, should help you understand why *caring* sometimes gets overlooked and how to safeguard against this from happening to you. This book is meant for anyone entering or already working in healthcare. While *Dignity in Care* was written to benefit patients and how you care for them—perhaps more to the point, how you care *about* them—it might also help you connect or reconnect with why you chose to work in healthcare in the first place. Sir William Osler, frequently described as the father of modern medicine said, "the good physician treats the disease; the great physician treats the patient who has the disease." *Dignity in Care* explores ways in which you can treat the patient and not lose sight of who they really are. Your work requires certain technical competencies and being able to carry out various assigned tasks. But real success requires so much more. After all, *patients are people with feelings that matter*.

References

1. Federman, D. ABC Nightline: "A lesson in patients." Aired Friday May 5, 2000. Transcript item number N000505. Information can be found at ABCNewsstore.com, or 1-800-callABC.
2. Chochinov HM. The secret is out: Patients are people with feelings that matter. Palliat Support Care. 2013;11:287–288.

When You Come Into My Room

When you come into my hospital room,
you need to know the facts of my life
that there is information not contained in my hospital chart
that I am 40 years married, with 4 children and 4 grandchildren
that I am "genetically Lutheran" ... with gut disease, like Luther himself
that I am a professor
that I teach teachers, priests, sisters how to nurture faith in the next generation
that I love earthy sensuous life, beauty, travel, eating, drinking J&B scotch, the
    theater, opera, the Chicago Symphony, movies, all kinds, water skiing, tennis,
    running, walking, camping
that I love loving, the wonder and awe of sexual intimacy
that I enjoy gardening, smell of soil in misty rain and scorching sun
that I have led a chronic illness group for 12 years

When You come into my room,
you need to know the losses of my life
that I have Crohn's disease and 3 small-bowel resections
that I have been hospitalized more than a dozen times for partial bowel obstruction
that I am chronically ill, and am seeking healing, not cure
that my disease has narrowed my life, constricted it
that I once fantasized but no longer dream about being president of Concordia or
    Mundelein College
that I can no longer eat fresh salads or drink a glass of wine
that I love teaching but sometimes have no energy left at the end of the day
that my Crohn's disease is active in the fall and spring, cyclically in tune with my work
that when I was to give my presidential address to the Association of Professors and
    Researchers in Religious Education, I was in the hospital for surgery
that when a colleague read my speech, I felt professionally diminished
that I can travel only where there is modern technology . . . I need fiberoptic
    intubation

When You come into my room,

you need to know my body

that I am afraid of medical procedures done at night . . . I awake fearfully to 10 feet of
air in an IV tube . . . I kink the tube and call . . . nurses come quickly . . . but I will
not forget . . . and my body remains sleepless in any hospital

that I know the loss of 25 pounds, not recorded in my chart . . . I had to beg for a
subclavian catheter for additional nutrition before I received one

that I am afraid of fifth-year residents . . . they tell me if my intestine does not open
in 4 more days, I will have to have another surgery . . . information not helpful
or useful

that I am on Pentasa, prednisone, Bentyl, Questran, vitamin B12, Relafen . . . more
than 20 pills each day . . . if I remember

that I hate rounds held outside my room, rounds that do not include nurses, my wife,
my children, my pastor, or even me . . . rounds done over me, around me, but not
with me

that this body seems battered, old, vulnerable, tired . . . but still me

that I live by medication

that I live by technology

that I live by waiting, in the eternal "advent season" of doctors' offices

When You come into my room,

you need to know my heart

that I am emotional . . . a fully functioning feeling person

that I am afraid of the NG tube, sometimes wrapped in my mouth, clogged

that I fear surgery, each time that I once felt I could not breathe in recovery

that I fear awakening from surgery with an ostomy

that with each partial obstruction I am anxious about another surgery

that I have lost confidence in my body

that I experience sadness and depression more often now than before the disease

that many persons chronically ill consider suicide, I am one of them

that the advent of symptoms is scary and debilitating

that I am angry at life's unfairness: my brother, older, eats too much drinks too much
plays too much and is healthy, always healthy so too my wife and it seems also
my colleagues . . . like I once was but am no longer, ever

that I worry about the future . . . insurance

that I am anxious about aging and how I will cope

that I long for one perfect day, only one symptom-free 24 hours
that I lust for remission
that being sick is narcissistic, boring, dull, painful
that there are times I want to give up

When You come into my room,
you need to know my mind and my spirit
that I seek meaning in suffering that suffering is the nudge to the religious question
that I have faith and lose it that I cling to my faith in spite of all evidence opposite
that I am trapped by the struggle for meaning yet engaged by it
that I am slowly coming to believe
that meaning is what we bring to suffering, not what we gain from it
that God, faith, meaning, ultimate concern, love, salvation are the being of my being
that I struggle with God
that Job was more just than God
that in my religious quest words are important, music is a mirror to my soul, and
      Eucharist, the stuff of mystery
that I believe deeply
that I need to engage suffering
that disease forces the God question and nurtures the Godless response that illness
      focuses the issue of death

When You come into my room,
you need to sustain my hope You need to know
that I believe love wins over hate, hope over despair, life over death
that I hope against hope
that I pray and believe prayer heals
that some days I am able to make meaning of suffering
that I am more gentle, more compassionate, better with dying, more loving, more
      sensitive, deeper in grief and in joy
Sit at my "mourning bench" if you are my physician listen to me, talk truthfully to me
you need to know all this if you want to heal me
And bear my rage about my disease
that I will never be cured
that my daughter has Crohn's disease and is only 33 years old that she too has had
      her first surgery and lives with many of my feelings and I am angry and sad
And support my hope that tomorrow there may be new medicines
that today you care deeply
that you will do your best

When you come into my hospital room,
promise me presence
promise me a healing partnership
keep hope alive
it is all I have.

—Schmidt SA. When you come into my room.
JAMA. 1996;276(7):512. doi:10.1001/jama.1996.03540070008002

1
Understanding Patienthood

Learning about dignity in care requires a deep understanding of what it feels like to be a patient. To really grasp this, start by looking into a mirror. What you will see is someone who shares the same vulnerabilities, risks, and uncertainties as your patients. A jarring thought perhaps, meant to highlight that in some very fundamental ways we are not so different from those we care for. On a day-to-day basis, those seeming differences surround and insulate us. Our patients are sick, we are not. Our patients are needy, we are not. Our patients must submit to assorted tests and poking and prodding of various kinds, while we are spared those indignities. Our patients may wear hospital gowns, while we don our white coats or hospital scrubs. Our patients are often afraid, anxious, vulnerable, and uncertain. We, on the other hand, can focus with objectivity, clarity, and purpose, on the specific clinical tasks at hand.

If you look more closely into the mirror you might consider that the eyes staring back at you may one day strain to see or the ears that could once hear a pin drop may eventually lose their acuity. The person whose reflection you see, no doubt, has a mind capable of grasping various facts, mastering certain tasks, and thinking through a multitude of problems and challenges. But people are vulnerable. Minds can become clouded with worry or depression or despair. Sickness or age or calamity can claim vitality, mobility, and mental clarity, and ultimately, will claim life itself. There are absolutely no exceptions to this rule. The reality of our own frailty is not something most of us keep top of mind, and why should we? Which is why, when catching our reflection in the mirror, we typically straighten our hair, perhaps apply makeup, or just make sure that we look presentable enough to get on with the rest of our day.

Occasionally we are reminded that, like our patients, we, too, are vulnerable. A young psychiatric resident lamented to her supervisor that she felt guilty each time she visited her sick and dying patient, a young man with AIDS-related complications who was quickly running out of therapeutic options and time. When her supervisor asked why this made her feel guilty, she responded that, unlike her patient, she could leave the hospital each day, enjoy being with her many friends and family, and anticipate a future filled with so much love and promise. In response she was offered what can only be described as stark and cold comfort. "Don't feel guilty," he told her, "one day it will be your turn to be sick and dying."

Existential Tap

Everyone experiences an occasional *existential tap*, a reminder that we are fragile and vulnerable. I recall such an encounter with my friend and colleague, Dr. Jim Derksen. Born in 1947, Jim became disabled during the polio epidemic of 1953. Although a wheelchair user ever since, he abhors being referred to as *wheelchair-bound*. Based on the mobility it provides him, he prefers to describe himself as *wheelchair-liberated*. Much of his adult life has been devoted to disability rights, helping found the Council of Canadians with Disabilities and the Canadian Disability Rights Council and being instrumental in the entrenchment of disability rights within the Canadian Charter of Rights and Freedoms. Several years ago I had the privilege of collaborating with him on a study that examined issues related to vulnerability, disability, and palliative care. One day Jim coyly referred to me as a "TAB." I took the bait: "Jim, what exactly does that mean? T-A-B?" He replied, "temporarily able bodied." Tap. The message was blatantly clear. Each one of us is fragile and vulnerable.

For most people, entry into patienthood begins with the realization that whoever you are, however you see yourself, whatever you do, believe in or aspire to, you are your body. In that moment of realization comes an emerging awareness that something about your body has gone or may be going wrong. Whatever that something is will usually manifest by way of symptoms of some sort: pain, fever, bleeding, bruising, weakness, stiffness, dizziness, shortness of breath; a change in vision, hearing, thinking; finding a lump; and the list goes on, covering sundry ways that people suddenly or insidiously discover that they are inextricably contained within their bodies.

That we are our bodies should hardly come as a surprise. Each day we look after our bodies in various ways by attending to feeding, voiding, bathing, and dressing. A reminder that *you are your body* would hardly seem necessary. Along with having a body comes familiarity with how bodies behave, what they can do, how they respond to different experiences, and expectations regarding how they will continue to do so well into the future. Entry into patienthood begins with the realization that these expectations may fall short of past performance and that bodies can and do eventually falter.

In the Blink of an Eye

At my age, early into my seventh decade, I estimate that I have blinked about 250,000,000 times. Each one of those times has been what I can only describe as a *successful blink*. My eyelids spontaneously close shut and immediately re-open, their purpose in doing so having been fulfilled and vision, thankfully, still intact. My eyes have witnessed a lifetime of experiences, from the birth of my children to the death of people I loved dearly. They have seen things that are breathtakingly beautiful and attempted to grasp the enormity of unspeakable ugliness, be those manifestations of hatred, poverty, violence, or injustice. Eyes are our windows onto the world.

Of course, behind the scenes of each blink are things that most of us are oblivious to. Every blink releases tears into the eye and produces lubricating oil from sebaceous glands between each eyelash to keep the tears from evaporating too quickly and mucus for lubrication, so that tears adhere to the surface of the eyeball. These fluids help flush out dirt or any foreign object that might sneak past the eyelids. Despite these highly technical, vital functions behind the scenes, we blithely carry on, taking in every view life has to offer. Then one day something happened. Despite every previous successful blink, blink 250,000,001 was different. This particular blink, which as I recall started off perfectly normal, ended with a sudden marked blurriness in my left eye, along with eerie undulating black streaks further obstructing my vision. For so many years without fail, my experience of vision was entirely subjective, sensory, and reliable. My body was now reminding me that vision is based on objective, delicate physiological facts. My very capable and gracious ophthalmologist confirmed my body's not so subtle message: "The explanation," he said, "is you're getting older." As he explained to me, "with age, the vitreous gel that sits behind the lens deteriorates, pulling on the retina, causing it to tear, thus the sudden blurriness. If it tears along a retinal blood vessel, that can cause bleeding into the vitreous, hence the black streaks." Tap. I am my body. How utterly annoying.

Shaping Emotional Responses to Illness

How one reacts to becoming a patient depends on a multitude of factors. However, *for every bodily ailment a patient encounters, anticipate an emotional response*. These responses are shaped by the *specifics* of the healthcare concern, the associated *uncertainty* with what is happening, the *perceived threat* connected with this change, the *meaning* one ascribes to this change, and the *personal characteristics and circumstances* of the person entering patienthood (Box 1.1). The combination of these factors leads to individualized responses, so a high degree of variability is to be expected.

Returning to my retinal tear by way of example, the specific symptoms are as I described them. In terms of uncertainty, without having an exact explanation for this sudden change, it was impossible to predict how this episode would play out, whether my vision would continue to deteriorate, whether these changes were reversible, or whether permanent and complete loss of vision in that eye was a possibility. Not knowing what to expect can elicit fear and anxiety. The trepidation of what might happen can often be as difficult to tolerate or cope with as the certainty of what will happen, even if that certainty points toward a difficult future course.

As for perceived threat, I knew my change in vision was not life-threatening. However, vision enables so many things that we take for granted, and the meaning we ascribe to those things further shapes our response. For instance, getting myself to the ophthalmologist. Suddenly the autonomy of being able to drive and go where I please was immediately replaced by the need to be driven. This sudden imposed dependency felt awkward, a disruption of a long-held assumption that being the person in the driver's seat was somehow immutable. Illness takes us out of the driver's seat. For an academic, vision has profound meaning given that the ability to read is closely rivaled by the ability to breathe. For me, reading fulfills an array of intellectual, emotional, and spiritual needs. It allows me to access a universe of information, ideas, insights, wisdom, vicarious experiences and emotions, and not infrequent inspiration, without which, it is hard to imagine still being me. Once the diagnosis was established (a retinal tear) and the remedy applied (laser surgery), the hardest part of my adjustment was not being able to read for 3 weeks. My physician was aware that this would be a difficult, but nevertheless, held firm: "You need to rest your eyes."

Box 1.1 Understanding Emotional Responses to Patienthood

- Specifics of the healthcare ailment or concern
- Uncertainty of what is happening
- Perceived bodily threat
- Meaning one ascribes to this change
- Personal characteristics and circumstances

Besides understanding the uncertainty of what is happening and the perceived threat and meaning one ascribes to those changes, it is critical to factor in the multiple personal characteristics and circumstances that are unique to each individual. Where is this person within the arc of their life story? What is their capacity to appreciate what is happening to them? What emotional reservoir are they able to tap into to cope with this particular challenge? Where or from whom do they draw strength and support? My personal circumstances and characteristics shaped my response to this health crisis in ways that are unique to me. I am old enough to have experienced other health challenges, so as annoying as the reminder that *I am my body* might have been, my adolescent self would have struggled far more with the existential shock of discovering I am not omnipotent. I have a job and sufficient financial security to be able to tolerate not working, or only partially working, for the duration of my recovery. I am also lucky enough to have wonderful people in my life, a loving wife and children, family, friends, and colleagues, all of whom in their own unique way value me, affirming that *you still matter, you are still you*, even though one of your primary expressions of self has been temporarily put on hold.

Of course, the template of response to patienthood (Box 1.1) depends on consciousness and the capacity to process whatever bodily events are occurring. There are instances when this is simply not possible; for example, a newborn or infant or someone whose cognition is temporarily or permanently failing in some way. Although this fundamentally alters the ability to perceive change, articulate uncertainty, or ascribe meaning, this template can be used to appreciate the responses of those who accompany patients into these healthcare experiences. While her 58-year-old sister Norma entered her second week in intensive care, Jackie struggled to make sense of this living nightmare. Norma was the eldest of three children and someone Jackie had always looked up to as a confidant and role model. How a previously healthy, beautiful, and vibrant person could suddenly now be unconscious, ventilator-dependent, and teetering between life and death was incomprehensible. Each day intensivists grappled to determine the *specific nature* of Norma's condition, at best only being able to rule out what it was not. The *uncertainty* of a diagnosis, along with the ruthlessness of her affliction, made Norma's bedside vigil even more excruciating. With each setback, Jackie and her family struggled to maintain hope while preparing for the worst. Daily reports, while offered in terms of respiratory status and various blood-related metrics, underscored the ominous *perceived bodily threat*, with the dawning realization that her illness was gaining the upper hand. Jackie also found herself contemplating what losing Norma *would mean* for her and her family, including her other sisters, aging parents, nieces, nephews, countless friends, and colleagues. This community of love and connection, leaning on and supporting one another, helped buoy them through their darkest days, no doubt extending beyond Norma's death and into their bereavement.

To summarize, unpacking emotional responses to entering patienthood is comprised of the follow key elements:

1. Patienthood starts with a reminder that you are your body.
2. Bodily ailments are accompanied by emotional responses.
3. To understand how patients respond to how their bodies are behaving or misbehaving, you must know:
    a. The specifics of the healthcare ailment or concern;
    b. The associated uncertainty of what is happening;
    c. The perceived threat;
    d. The meaning one ascribes to these changes;
    e. The personal characteristics and circumstances of the individual now entering patienthood.

Understanding Emotional Responses to Patienthood: A Case Example

Until being diagnosed with head and neck cancer at the age of 67 years, Jacques was a content and successful symphony violaist. Following the discovery of a tumor at the back of his tongue, he underwent major surgery, extensive neck dissection, removal of significant portions of his tongue, and skin grafting, followed by a slow and difficult recovery. The previously described template provides a means of deconstructing Jacques's response to becoming a patient.

You are your body: The back of the tongue usually demands little if any attention. It contributes to the process of swallowing, the ability to taste, and plays a role in being able to articulate and speak. Jacques was a man of refined tastes. He delighted in good food, good wine, and good conversation, especially when that included female companionship. He saw these indulgences as a perfect counterpoint to his life as a professional musician and ones that he approached with genuine reverence and a hardy appetite. His first indication that something was wrong included inexplicable pain at the back of his mouth and occasionally spitting up blood. There was nothing subtle about this particular existential tap. With persistent symptoms and escalating discomfort came the realization that his tongue, a silent player up until now, was about to rudely insist on taking center stage.

Bodily ailments are accompanied by emotional responses: In Jacques's case, of this there could be no doubt. He was a man who felt emotions deeply and intensely and, as a musician and artist, was someone whose ability to feel and show passion were second nature. In response to his diagnosis, he expressed fear, anxiety, depression, and disappointment for all the ways that cancer threatened to disrupt his various cherished plans and a deep, soul-crushing grief. Jacques wore his heart on his sleeve, unashamedly and without inhibition. This was not a matter of personal choice, nor was he conflicted about it. Quite simply, this was who he was.

Not everyone has this kind of emotional repertoire. Some people are more stoic than others and attempt, to varying degrees, to suppress their feelings, frightened of their possible responses as much as they are of whatever malady is brewing inside of them. For some people, allowing feelings to surface or take expression can be cathartic, liberating and even healing. For others, it can evoke feelings of fragility and heightened exposure. It is one thing to feel as though you are coming undone, but quite another to let others into that terrifying reality. While Jacques was completely transparent in his responses, others work hard to repress or hide their feelings. For those patients, *keeping it together* means not letting others see that their sense of self and perceived competence is starting to unravel.

The specifics of the healthcare ailment or concern: The presentation of tongue cancer leaves little doubt that your body is insisting on becoming the center of attention. This is no simple *tap*, but metaphorically more akin to an existential slap across the face. Among other things, patients with tongue cancer may experience pain, weight loss, difficulty or painful swallowing, spitting up blood, hoarseness, or problems with articulation. The back of Jacques's tongue was no longer some hidden and silent part of his anatomy. By the time he sought medical care, Jacques's tongue had managed to capture his full and complete attention.

The uncertainty of what is happening: A diagnosis of cancer is frightening to anyone, and Jacques was no exception. The uncertainties of illness had been discussed with him, and he had been told that the likelihood of living more than 5 years was about 50-50. He was no doubt informed that his chances largely depended on the type and stage of his cancer and that with aggressive treatment, there were risks, including facial disfigurement, radiation effects such as dry mouth and difficulties swallowing, and, of course, the possibility that his cancer could spread.

The perceived threat: For most people, a diagnosis of cancer is synonymous with a death sentence; at the very least, people associate cancer with the possibility that they may die. Of course, there are many kinds of cancers with widely varying prognoses. Jacques worried about death, but, far more so, he worried about cancer threatening the things he held dear in life. Of course, there was his music, his plans to perform various concerts, organize several music competitions, and nurture young, up-and-coming musicians. He had been a strikingly handsome man. Seeing him in concert, I recall him exuding confidence, even swagger, with his dark hair slicked back and his viola resting easily on his shoulder. For patients with head and neck cancer, sense of self can be particularly vulnerable. The human face, more so than anything else about us, distinguishes who we are, how we are identified, and the image people conjure in their mind's eye when they think of us. While the face is no more the person than the cover is the book, it happens to be the cover on display in every human encounter. A sudden threat or change in appearance is tantamount to an assault on the very essence of who we are.

The meaning one ascribes to this change: To understand Jacques, one needs to understand the centrality of music—listening to music, teaching music, performing music, and promoting music—in his life. Music was the center of his universe. When complications secondary to treatment prevented him from playing, his world began to quickly crumble. When he contemplated having to place his viola in storage for safekeeping, our conversation took on the quality of planning a funeral. Around that time, he shared a particular conversation he had had with his medical oncologist. According to his doctor, based on the objective medical evidence, scans, pathology reports, blood work, and the like, things were looking better. In fact, he told me his oncologist said he might look forward to a good quality of life. Jacques's retort, given his inability to play music was, "what life?"

Personal characteristics and circumstances to be considered: By his own admission, Jacques had placed all his eggs in one basket, and that basket was his music. Up until now, well into his seventh decade, this had served him quite well. Music had been his ticket out of his previous life in Eastern Europe and, upon arriving in Canada, had provided him a vocation that had taken him around the world. But his devotion to music had preempted other choices and opportunities he might otherwise have considered. And so, when his cancer returned and he was no longer able to play and his fate with advancing disease appeared to be sealed, he reflected on the consequences of those choices, the absence of family or anyone who would care or even take notice of his absence. I remember him sitting in my office one day, reflecting on the sad truth that there was no one in the waiting room or at home anxiously anticipating his return or wondering how his appointment had gone. All that awaited him was an empty apartment, where even the classical music radio station was starting to feel like a painful reminder of something he had been forced to leave behind.

Patienthood, Personhood and a Revised Sense of Self

Becoming a patient is a transformative experience, particularly when it challenges our previously held assumptions about who we are. It is deeply ironic that although all of healthcare is organized around looking after patients, no one really wants to *just* be a patient. Entering patienthood means confronting a broader realization of what it means to be human. Becoming a patient means facing vulnerability, dependency, and uncertainty and moreover discovering that those are all within our personal repertoire. In our state of wellness, we assume that being strong, independent, and in control are the norm. Whether it arrives by way of sickness, injury, or life experience, everyone eventually comes to know that being human limits and challenges those fleeting assumptions.

Depending on when and how it arrives, patienthood can disrupt our previous sense of self. Sometimes this disruption can be subtle, little more than an underlying existential dis-ease, leaving us feeling less certain than we felt before. At other times, it can be earth-shattering. Like someone who has been assaulted, patients can be left feeling that life is less safe, that our ability to stave off bad things is less certain, and the mantra "things will be ok" is more a plaintive wish than a firmly held belief. Of course, the quality and nature of this disruption will depend on the specifics of the patient encounter and how an individual responds to those circumstances (as described in Box 1.1). Generally minor encounters yield mild disruptions. While my retinal tear was upsetting and temporarily inconvenient, my physical and psychological recovery was for the most part uncomplicated and complete. My awareness of aging is ubiquitous, albeit subtle, and this experience has not left me worried about the outcome of each subsequent blink.

Other encounters with patienthood can be more traumatizing and have lingering effects. Take the case of a patient who battled a soul-crushing depression. Until then this middle-aged married man and father of three children had been a highly successful architect. He was earning a very comfortable living and his children seemed well settled into school, jobs, and relationships, when, suddenly by his account, things started to turn dark. At first he noticed trouble concentrating. Then his sleep became disrupted, and his appetite virtually disappeared. Over a course of several weeks, he went from feeling relatively content with his life to no longer being able to experience pleasure or joy whatsoever. The future looked utterly bleak and without promise. When he was not battling overwhelming anxiety, he was struggling to stave off feelings of failure, inadequacy, and hopelessness. Life no longer seemed worth living, and thoughts of suicide were never far from consideration. While he responded to treatment over the course of several months, seemingly making a full recovery, he was left with residual scarring that altered his prior sense of self. He felt less sure of himself, less confident that he would always be able to provide for his family or that he would always somehow manage to land on his feet. Up until now he was convinced that his own resilience, fortitude, and ingenuity would always see him through. He felt as if he had been kidnapped by his depression and psychologically held hostage, kept at bay from his family, friends, and all he held dear. While he was no longer depressed, the experience of having been depressed changed his worldview, which was now tainted by a sense of his own fragility and fallibility.

Being a patient changes people. Patienthood happens to persons and imposes a reality that no one wants to face, that minds and bodies are imperfect and can fail, and, depending on the proclivities of any given ailment at any given time, autonomy and the ability to fend for ourselves and land on our feet is far from assured. For the person confronting this universal reality, this can come as a life-altering shock. However, within the context of the human condition, these encounters are commonplace. While who you are as a person defies measure and is entirely unique, who you are as a patient and the ways in which minds and bodies impose limitations, sickness, and affliction implicates physical elements of your being that are generic, objective, and physiologically predictable.

Not Just a Patient

The term "patient" denotes someone with generic and objective features which usually fall under a collective label (cardiac patients, cancer patients, respiratory patients, stroke patients, and so on). A dialysis nurse once told me that her job had become so technical, it was hard not to think of patients as "kidneys on legs." In other words, her perception was consistent with the notion that *patients are their bodies.* Healthcare providers are tasked with determining how bodies go wrong. They undertake various tests and tasks to arrive at a *diagnosis*, a word that comes from the Greek *dia* meaning *a part*, and *gignoskein*, meaning *to know.* To make a diagnosis is to know the patient, that is to know *a part* of the patient, based on his or her particular ailment. But recall *patients are people with feelings that matter*. While the patient presents with a complaint or symptom that implicates the body, patients are people, and understanding feelings that a given healthcare encounter may trigger falls within the purview of any professional caregiver wanting to achieve dignity in care.

People do not easily integrate patient-acquired insights or bodily disruptions into their overall sense of self. My erstwhile depressed patient recoiled at the notion of somehow being weak or less capable. And yet, despite wishing it were otherwise, he seemed unable to shake a feeling of heightened susceptibility. The internal safety net he once assumed would always be there to catch him, his sense of self-efficacy, turned out to be fallible and capable of tearing. Over the years this has turned into a wistful recognition, some might call it wisdom, that fragility is a form of residual emotional scarring. Rather than viewing his depression solely in terms of individual fallibility, he has come to appreciate that vulnerability is woven into the universal fabric of the human condition.

The word "disease" has French roots dating back to the early 14th century, meaning discomfort, inconvenience, distress, or trouble. The Old French *desaise* combines *des*, meaning *without*, and *aise* meaning *ease*. Being a patient means living without ease, hence dis-ease. The interplay between how we define ourselves as persons and how we experience patienthood provides important insights into how people respond to disease, disability, and dependence on healthcare. It is hard to integrate the experience of being sick into our sense of self. *Illness may happen to me*, but I loathe the idea that it threatens to define me. And the sicker you are and the more protracted the experience of dis-ease, the more likely that illness leaves an existential, psychological, or spiritual imprint. And as most patients soon discover, sickness is a cruel but compelling teacher.

Disability offers a profound vantage point to understand the integration of disease, personhood, and an emerging sense of self. As Catherine Frazee, disability rights activist and scholar so aptly put it, "while disabled people are unique, unusual and even at times extraordinary, we are not the other— falling short of some unspoken threshold. We are fully human—complete, complex and undiminished."[1] In other words, disability is not synonymous with fractured personhood, despite widely held biases and assumptions to the contrary. Bodies, all bodies, can and will behave at odds with our preconceived notions of normality. It could be argued that deviations are the norm and the idea of *normal* is illusory. Patients must accommodate to their specific bodily variations in the service of establishing or maintaining an integrated and intact sense of self. Failure to do so, wherein patients feel defined by their ailment or disability, can lead to suffering and a distorted or constricted sense of who they are as a person.

Resistance to Patienthood

The interplay between patienthood and personhood, and the degree to which they shape and impact one another, determines an emerging, integrated sense of self (see Table 1.1). The quest to maintain personhood will usually include some form of resistance, staving off the imposition and existential assault of becoming a patient. Resistance of some sort, even subtle resistance, is a way for patients to express their unwillingness to be defined based on their disease or disability.

Jacques railed against cancer and craved recognition as the creative and artistic soul he had always been, not simply *the patient* he sensed himself becoming. He had always had a commanding presence. As an audience member—long before he was ill and became my patient—I recall seeing him on the stage, looking suave, debonair, and completely comfortable in his orchestral role. Little surprise that his resistance had a prominent musical theme. He invariably arrived at appointments carrying what I thought of as his personal talisman, an old beat-up leather valise, chock-full of music and brochures describing various local, national, and international recitals. Despite weather conditions, good or bad, he always wore white cotton gloves to protect his fingers. One way of coaxing him out of the psychological doldrums that threatened to envelop him was listening, listening with genuine interest, curiosity, and appreciation, to him talk about music, musicians, concerts, tours, and conductors. For Jacques, being listened to was a way of affirming who he was despite the unrelenting encroachment of his advancing cancer. While struggling with postsurgical complications, mouth pain, drooling, difficulty

Table 1.1 Sense of self and features of personhood/patienthood

Integrated sense of self	
Personhood	Patienthood
Strength and resilience	Vulnerability
Independence, autonomy, self-reliant	Dependency, reliance on others
Being in control	Relinquishing control
Individual	Generic
You are more than your body	You are your body

swallowing, and weight loss, he seemed to redouble his efforts to stave off patienthood by trying to organize musical competitions and festivals, arranging everything from venues to prize money. While cancer did everything it could to take the upper hand, Jacques fought mightily to keep music where it had always been in his life, front and center stage.

Waiting rooms are a good place to observe resistance to patienthood being played out. At its most understated, resistance looks and feels like annoyance or impatience. People may be pacing, others may be at the reception desk asking if they will be seen anytime soon. Every person there has had to relinquish his or her schedule for the sake of getting help. Feeling or acting annoyed or impatient is a way of asserting, "my time matters; I don't really want to be here. I have other things I would rather be doing."

These feelings are natural given that most of us like to be in charge of our lives. Many people, especially those who are naïve to the experience of disease or disability, consider autonomy to be synonymous with personhood. Patienthood imposes the realization that autonomy and control, like our state of health, is fragile and can be temporarily fleeting or permanently altered or compromised. Just ask these people in the waiting room. Each of them is having their *TAB moment*. We are all temporarily able-bodied. Any of them will tell you: if they were truly in charge, they would rather be elsewhere.

The last time I wandered through one of our hospital waiting areas I noticed various forms of resistance being played out. Many people were on their smart phones, surfing the net or texting. While I do not know what they were saying, the subtext was easy to infer: "I am a person who likes having access to information. I am someone with connections to other people. My life is out there, not in here." Some were with relatives or friends, some chatting, others not. Several seemed reasonably distracted by a televised hockey game, even though our home team was not playing. Others were reading books they had the foresight to bring with them or whatever old magazines happened to be lying around. Each was expressing a form of resistance by not allowing some aspect of who they are—someone who reads, someone who likes hockey, someone who is connected to friends and family—to succumb to patienthood. *I am not my illness, or my ailing body part. Don't define me as such.*

I did notice one young man off in the corner of the waiting area, his head hung down between his knees, not interacting with anyone, not moving a great deal, silent. While I suppose he may have drifted off to sleep, certainly one way of temporarily disconnecting from an illness experience, his posture suggested otherwise. I sensed he was uncomfortable and trying to retreat somewhere within the deep recesses of his mind, where, if he tried hard enough, pain and sickness might not touch him. Illness and despair, however, have a frightening reach. Sometimes resistance is little more than a remote, internal voice telling us to *just breathe*, to not let ourselves be consumed by something that threatens to swallow us whole. The silent, hunched-over young man in the corner of the waiting room reminded me that resistance is not infallible and, until the threat subsides, can only partially stave off the inevitable vulnerability and fear that follows in its wake.

My friend Jim Derksen is an expert at resistance. He always wears a bright African moo-moo dress, which he told me serves a dual purpose. As a wheelchair user, he finds moo-moos are extremely convenient and don't require having to coax uncooperative limbs into a more traditional shirt and pants. Jim also knows this garb defines his look and draws attention away from him being seen *just* as a wheelchair user. Add to that a long gray beard, ponytail, and colorful tam to complete the mental image. Jim's form of resistance essentially says, "I refuse to be seen or defined based on my disability." Occasionally having young children mistake him for Santa Claus speaks to the success of his unique strategy.

Trust and the Entry into Patienthood

The word "vulnerable" comes from the Latin *vulnerare*, meaning *to wound* or *to pluck or tear*. There is something about the experience of patienthood that threatens to wound, pluck, or tear at our sense of self. It confronts our feeling of intactness by revealing we are capable of tearing and limits our autonomy and ability by way of imposing dependency and disability. Feeling vulnerable is a profound and universal experience, forcing us to surrender to the will of our bodies while deferring to others to get care. This is not easy for patients as it requires trusting someone to address needs that can no longer be independently met or managed.

For those entering care, it is the experience of being *cared for* that fosters the emergence of trust. Hence, healthcare providers must recognize and respond to patients' vulnerability if they are to gain their trust.[2] A systematic review of cancer patients' trust in their physician reported that while trust was partially based on a sense of technical competence, it was also gauged by perceived honesty, patient-centered communication, and organization in the clinical setting. Trust in physicians is associated with real and tangible patient benefits, such as decreased fear and distress and lower perceived risk. It also results in more confidence in medical decision-making, less likelihood of seeking a second opinion, and adherence to medical advice.[3] One study on the longitudinal effects of trust and decision-making preferences on diabetic patients reported that trust was positively related to blood sugar control, physical health–related quality of life, and satisfaction with care.[4]

Trust is not a one-size-fits-all endeavor. Life shapes us in different ways and, accordingly, determines our capacity to trust. Those who have encountered disloyalty, betrayal, hurt, and disappointment in life are less inclined to see the world as beneficent and trustworthy. On the other hand, people who have experienced love, dependability, and fulfillment are more apt to be trusting despite the associated risks. Each clinical encounter has its own tempo, with some providing the opportunity to develop trust over time. Early in my psychiatric residency, a severely traumatized, sexually abused young woman was assigned to my care. She desperately wanted help managing her life that was rapidly spinning out of control. The memory of her fear is as palpable today, decades later, as it was during those early sessions. She was afraid of me and, to be frank, given the enormity of her anguish, my lack of experience and the apparent damage inflicted by years of abuse and violence, I was afraid of her and her potential for self-harm. My supervisor encouraged patience, assuring me that time, compassion, listening, and having her experience a relationship with a male that was not abusive or distorted by self-serving motivation might eventually yield therapeutic benefits. And, just as he predicted, both our fears eventually dissipated, making way for trust and slow but steady healing.

In many clinical encounters, trust emerges to a very different tempo. Something happens that abruptly hurls someone into needing medical attention. Unlike other chance meetings, which may or may not go well or can easily be forgotten or written off, this encounter is different. After all, treatment, recovery, or at the very least an explanation of what has gone wrong hangs in the balance. The margin for error is thin, and there is little room to negotiate terms. The patient needs help now, and your role is to deliver it. At times like these, trust is not a slow and gentle negotiation. Instead, it is an assumption that those who want help will attempt to make, placing themselves utterly and completely in the hands of a typically unknown healthcare professional. That is the quandary that patients find themselves in. This is no party game where you are asked to close your eyes and fall backward into the arms of the person standing behind you. While you can always bow out of that harmless game of trust, entering healthcare leaves you nowhere else to go. Most patients do so with hope and trepidation and, depending on their ability to trust, a combination of resentment, faith, fear, and resignation. "Will the person at triage see more than my desperation and neediness? Will the nurses and doctors examining my body do so with professionalism, kindness, and respect?" Unlike a game of trust, there is no option to turn around, look into the eyes of the person you are being asked to trust, and size them up. And so, while not knowing with certainly if those arms are strong enough, capable enough, or willing enough to catch them, most people just let themselves fall.

Even when patients are metaphorically caught—that is, the right diagnosis is made, an accurate explanation is found, the correct treatment is administered—the landing can still feel unacceptably rough, unless, as Anatole Broyard (see Box 1.2) said, there is some form of *acknowledgment*; acknowledgment that we are not simply what ails us, but individual, unique, valuable and valued, whole persons. "Why bother with sick people, why try to save them," Broyard said, "if they're not worth acknowledging? When a doctor refuses to acknowledge a patient, he is, in effect, abandoning him to his illness."[5]

And so, who are these people we call patients? They are anyone facing the realization, through personal experience, that minds and bodies are fallible. Through no fault of their own, they must now relinquish many of the privileges and benefits that go along with being completely healthy. They are people whose autonomy, temporarily or permanently, is compromised. For some, perhaps for the first time ever, dependency is the hard pill they are being

---

Box 1.2 From *Intoxicated by My Illness* by Anatole Broyard

Anatole Broyard[5] was a brilliant writer and the former editor of the *New York Times Book Reviews*. While living with prostate cancer, an illness that eventually claimed his life, Broyard wrote about his struggle not to be defined by the illness that was ravaging his body. While much of illness narrative has a similar purpose, it can often be maudlin and depressing. Broyard, on the other hand, wrote with a unique and compelling voice. "Writing," he said, "is a counterpoint to my illness. It forces the cancer to go through my character before it can get to me." He had a ribald sense of humor and an eye for the profound and the absurd.

The doctor warned me that, like radiation, hormonal manipulations would kill my libido. I find this hard to believe, especially in the case of a writer, for whom sexuality is inseparable from consciousness. After three months of treatment this has not yet happened, and I persist in believing that it won't. I've been manipulating my sexual hormones all my life, and I don't see how a drug can deprive me of this privilege. My libido is lodged not only in my prostate, but in my imagination, my memory, my conception of myself, my appreciation of women and of life itself. It belongs as much to my identity and my aesthetics as it does to physiology. When the cancer threatened my sexuality, my mind became immediately erect.

forced to swallow. Little wonder they are frightened, irritated, expectant, and perhaps even embarrassed about the physical and psychological exposure they must now endure. Ask any of them and they will tell you that they desperately want to be seen as the person they have always been. Given the chance they would remind you that they are someone's child, parent, partner, companion, friend, or neighbor. Many might say that they love and are loved, that their lives have meaning and purpose. They now understand what health-care professionals must never forget: patients are people, and people can be wounded and torn. In that regard, patients are no different from those who care for them and into whose arms they are about to fall.

References

1. Frazee C. *Dispatches from disabled country: Selected writings by Catherine Frazee*. In press.
2. Clark CC. Trust in medicine. J Med Philosophy. 2002;27:11–29.
3. Hillen MA, de Haes HCJM, Smets EMA. Cancer patients' trust in their physician: A review. Psycho-Oncology. 2011;20:227–241.
4. Lee Y-Y, Lin JL. How much does trust really matter? A study of the longitudinal effects of trust and decision-making preferences on diabetic patient outcomes. Patient Educ Counsel. 2011;85:406–412.
5. Broyard A. *Intoxicated by my illness: And other writings on life and death*. Fawcett Columbine; 1992.

The Death of Ivan Ilyich

He saw that no one felt for him, because no one even wished to grasp his position. Only Gerasim recognized it and pitied him. And so Ivan Ilyich felt at ease only with him. He felt comforted when Gerasim supported his legs (sometimes all night long) and refused to go to bed, saying: "don't you worry, Ivan Ilyich. I'll get sleep enough later on," or when he suddenly became familiar and exclaimed: "If you weren't sick it would be another matter, but as it is, why should I grudge a little trouble?" Gerasim alone did not lie; everything showed that he alone understood the facts of the case and did not consider it necessary to disguise them, but simply felt sorry for his emaciated and enfeebled master. Once when Ivan Ilyich was sending him away he even said straight out: "We shall all of us die, so why should I grudge a little trouble?"— expressing the fact that he did not think his work burdensome, because he was doing it for a dying man and hoped someone would do the same for him when his time came.

—Leo Tolstoy

2

The ABCDs of Dignity-Conserving Care

Let's Start at the Very Beginning, a Very Good Place to Start

> Nobody cares how much you know, until they know how much you care.
> —**Theodore Roosevelt**

By now it should be clear that understanding patient experience requires an appreciation that patienthood implicates whole persons. While patienthood is usually described in terms of specific ailments or symptoms, whole persons can only be fully understood when their collective physical, psychological, existential, and spiritual dimensions are taken into account. Jill Taylor-Brown is a retired social worker and former Head of the Department of Patient and Family Support Services at CancerCare Manitoba. Her career in oncology spanned several decades, and she carries with her deep wisdom and countless stories. She says that "understanding patients means understanding complete and complex human beings, and all of the people that love and care about them and this complex network of connections. There are times where the patient in healthcare is invisible; it's like they have become an inanimate object, present but not really seen. This is especially important for healing, particularly when we are thinking about people who are living with long term chronic illness or are nearing end-of-life. How can you heal if you are being treated by a healthcare team that doesn't see all of you?" She recalled a patient who told her, "I wish that when I go to see the oncologist, I could take everybody with me who loves and cares about me and that all of us could be in the room. Then she could see how important it is that how she takes care of me is impacting all of the people that I love and care for."

Being *seen*, which implicates being familiar with the intricacies of patienthood and personhood, is key to understanding, unraveling, and contextualizing how people respond to disease and the need for healthcare. Without this perspective and insight, healthcare providers will strive to meet the needs of patients and families without really appreciating the delicate and complex landscape they are trying to navigate. Little wonder that, despite good intentions, when it comes to providing dignity in care, healthcare professionals can sometimes find themselves wandering aimlessly, feeling frustrated and often lost.

Tom Roche was a highly respected social worker at CancerCare Manitoba who sadly died of cancer in February 2019. He was known for his storytelling, compassion, and gentle wisdom. He recalled a patient "who was in his early fifties and had mutiple myloma. He was so put off by the initial interactions he was having with his physician, he was thinking, 'I'd rather just suffer with this condition than go through the inhuman experience of being treated like a number. It's just not worth it.' I recall him saying that he felt he was not being looked at. 'It's like here is the chart and the chart and computer were the focus of attention.' So there was a sense that his anxiety was not being talked about; I really don't see you, I'm literally not looking at you. There is this perception that I don't want to answer any of your questions that you may have about what might happen, or what you can expect or how to understand any of this. So again, there was this sense of being dismissed, which was incredibly difficult for the patient and his wife."

In reflecting on dignity in care, Dr. Joel Gingerich, a young medical oncologist specializing in genitourinary cancers and palliative care observed that "physical symptoms are the area where we get the most training, but that makes up only a portion of what patients are going through, maybe only 50%. There are a lot of other areas that are not looked at as much and we hardly get any training. But attending to the whole person makes such a difference, paying attention to the psychosocial, the spiritual and existential parts of patient experience. I have to look at all of that, trying to incorporate the whole person into how I manage their symptoms or how I manage their cancer."

In reflecting on whole-person care, I recall visiting an elderly woman with an advanced gastrointestinal malignancy on the palliative care ward. She struck me as somber, based, I assumed, on her dire medical situation. As we began to talk, she indicated that she was really quite at peace with her pending death; that she had lived a good and long life and saw little tragedy in the fact that her life would soon come to an end. When asked to explain this apparent acceptance in contrast to her outward demeanor, her eyes welled up as she shared her source of as yet unspoken anguish. Her 50-year-old son was battling pancreatic cancer and was currently in another hospital dealing with his latest postsurgical complications. While she said her own death was easy to contemplate, his grim prognosis and the anguish of her daughter-in-law and their children triggered deep sorrow. In sharing her story, she proved that my initial assumptions about her sadness and its connection with her own illness were entirely wrong. Without taking the time to find out what was really going on, I suspect other healthcare providers might have made the same mistake. Tragically, while they might have genuinely tried to take care of her and respond to her various palliative care needs, they would have done so in the absence of having any idea who this patient really was.

Another patient I saw that day told a very different story, albeit offering a similar lesson. Mrs. F. was a 65-year-old married First Nations woman, now in hospital nearing the end of her long illness with metastatic breast cancer. When asked what I needed to know about her as a person to give her the best care possible, she disclosed that she had been a victim of the residential school system. These schools constitute a shameful chapter in Canadian history, wherein the Canadian government, working in conjunction with various Christian churches, funded a program that was specifically designed to remove First Nations, Métis, and Inuit children from the influence of their families and traditions in order to assimilate them into the dominant Canadian culture. Mrs. F. said that because of the residential school, she always had a hard time trusting people. She in fact moved 82 times so as not to let anyone get too close to her. While this had gotten better over time, she still struggled with being able to trust people. "People in white coats scare me," she said. And while she wished she could be more trusting, she confessed, "it is hard for me." She sometimes worried that she would not be told the whole truth or that people would see her as not being deserving of the whole truth. She appreciated people being friendly toward her but remained frightened of authority figures. "Authority scares me, but I'm not as bad as I used to be." Again, while it might be possible to provide her technical care in the absence of knowing her story and her fear, the cultural, historical, and emotional gap separating her and the next *whited-coated*, albeit good-intentioned healthcare provider might prove too vast to negotiate.

Core Competencies

While dignity in care requires a deep understanding of what influences patient experience, it is equally important to appreciate how the innate qualities and outlooks of healthcare providers shape the clinical encounter. Medicine prides itself on objectivity and its ability to create frameworks that enable practitioners to predict outcomes and determine best practices. That is why medicine is replete with models, formulas, care pathways, clinical guidelines, standards of practice, and the like, each of which point healthcare providers in very specific, logical directions. Ideally, any given problem or situation corresponds to a data-driven algorithm, enabling healthcare providers to understand, interpret, and respond to whatever problem or challenge they may be facing. Take for instance the ABCs of critical care. Anyone working in healthcare is expected to know and understand their ABCs: airway, breathing, and circulation. Healthcare providers of all stripes are expected to understand that if a patient is unconscious or unresponsive, they must check to see that the patient's airway is clear, establish that the patient is breathing, and determine if circulation has been compromised.

Frameworks such as the ABCs are intended to elicit distinct and effective responses and go hand in hand with certain corresponding obligations and responsibilities. By way of training, I am a psychiatrist. While my area of expertise is mental health, this does not absolve me of the responsibilities associated with being a healthcare professional. If I happen upon a patient who is unconscious or unresponsive and choose to walk away or fail to invoke the ABCs, I would be shirking my professional obligations. To claim that my area of expertise somehow protects me from having to maintain core professional competencies would, rightfully, garner little support. *The patient died, but I provided impeccable professional empathy*! Laughable for certain, and yet when it comes to the human side of care, healthcare professionals frequently argue this very line of defense: that is, it is not my responsibility.

If dignity in care is not included within core competencies, it is easy for healthcare professionals to claim their innocence in not providing or embracing these elements of care or more accurately, *caring*. Unless the requirements of dignity in care can be articulated and basic competencies identified, it is hard to hold healthcare professionals accountable. In an area of healthcare that has such a personal and lasting influence on patient experience, healthcare professionals can find themselves practicing in a vacuum, devoid of any real data, clear guidelines, or tangible expectations. In the absence of anything better, trainees or employees are often told *be a good person, trust your gut*. In many instances, even those rather tepid conversations do not occur. Instead, there is an assumption that people will somehow figure it out and behave accordingly. Ask any healthcare care administrator or patient representative; they will tell you that not every healthcare provider has a talented gut, that leaving people to simply follow their own devices and instincts, despite good intentions, does not always lead to good outcomes. Clearly, we need to do better. In the service of doing better, healthcare providers need to consider the *ABCDs of dignity-conserving care*, which define the core competencies of dignity in care. They are healthcare provider qualities and outlooks that shape every clinical encounter, and are, indeed, a very good place to start.

A Stands for Attitude

> We do not see things as they are. We see things as we are.
> —The Talmud

Understanding the core competencies of dignity in care begins in the same way this book began, and that is by looking in the mirror. Your attitude, the way you see and experience the world as filtered through your own biases, outlooks, beliefs, and assumptions, has a profound influence on patient experience and that of their families. Despite this sounding intuitive and vaguely pontifical, it is empirically driven. In a study of more than 200 terminally ill patients, our research group examined issues that feature prominently among people drawing closer to death.[1] Pain, nausea, shortness of breath, anxiety, depression, appetite, energy, sense of well-being, quality of life—in effect, we examined key variables that might influence end-of-life experience. The most revealing finding of this study was that the single most ardent predictor of patient dignity was *appearance* or, more to the point, how people perceived themselves to be seen.

Healthcare providers spend the entirety of their training learning things they need to know about and things they need to do with or for their patients. Our findings on the other hand indicate that, from a patient's perspective, the most important thing that influences something as vital as dignity is how their healthcare provider sees them, which of course depends on their attitude toward patients. Other research designed to look at associations between patient experience and sense of dignity toward the end of life yielded very similar results.[2] We gave patients with advanced cancer a list of items and asked which of them might influence their sense of dignity. Three-quarters of respondents said that *no longer feeling like the person I once was* would undermine their sense of dignity. This is a critical issue, given that the psychology of illness is the psychology of loss. The more illness undermines things we affiliate with a sense of self, the more dignity is likely to be compromised. The items most highly affiliated with sense of dignity were *feeling a burden to others* and *not feeling treated with respect*. Feeling like a burden has been identified in most studies examining interest in euthanasia or assisted suicide. People who contemplate death-hastening measures almost invariably report feeling a burden to others. It would seem that feeling a burden to others is the equivalent of existential extremis. To perceive oneself a burden means entering a mindset wherein you no longer feel you serve or have any meaningful purpose or function. To feel a burden means to believe that your very existence imposes a drain on others, one that far outweighs whatever benefits or contributions you are still capable of offering.

It is easy to imagine how burden to others is context-dependent. A wheelchair user, for instance, living in a third-floor suite, might feel like she is a burden to others should the elevator break down and require friends and family to carry her up and down many flights of stairs. Their attitude in doing so, whether they do so begrudgingly and with resentment or willingly, with understanding and empathy, will clearly influence the extent to which she starts to feel like a burden. Tiny subtleties can taint, or alternatively rescue, the experience. A frown, a lack of conversation, complaining about how much of an imposition this is, rough handling, or an abrupt departure; any of these might leave her feeling that, despite getting the help she needed, the existential price was exceedingly high in being made to feel little more than a dead weight to be moved from one place to another, a task indistinguishable from carrying a bag of cement or a sack of potatoes.

Rescue begins with the realization that *this weight* is by no means dead. A smile or perhaps words of shared frustration ("When is that landlord going to fix this elevator?!"), conversation that acknowledges something of who this person is ("What's your name? How long have you been living here? What have you been up to today?"), or sharing something of yourself ("My name is . . . you would not believe the day I've had. . . .") allows for a different kind of engagement, one that sees two people share in a genuine moment of connection. There is a kind of reciprocity in these connections that mitigates feelings of being a burden, wherein both parties can recognize personhood in the other. In the clinical arena, this kind of attitude includes an appreciation of *patient as person.*

A wonderful nurse I work with shared her story of one such connection, which took place during her own personal encounter with breast cancer. While nearly 20 years have passed since she was declared disease-free, there is a particular moment, she said, that is indelibly etched in her mind. As she was laying on a gurney, being rolled into the operating room by a patient transport clerk, he stopped to take a moment to look into her eyes from behind his mask, place his hand gently on her shoulder, and tell her "it is going to be ok." It was a brief instance of two human beings sharing a moment of mutual understanding, infused with pathos, trepidation, and hope.

Besides burden to others, study participants with advanced cancer indicated that *not being treated with respect* was equally likely to undermine their sense of dignity. Burden to others and not being treated with respect are two sides of the same existential coin. If feeling a burden to others means no longer believing one's very existence serves any purpose or has any meaning, then not feeling worthy of respect is a painful, albeit logical consequence. Respect, however, is something that healthcare providers can either confer or withhold from their patients. Respect, from the Latin *respectus*, means the *action of looking back*. How do we look back at our patients, and, in turn, how do they perceive our critical gaze? Do they sense our ability to see them as valuable, important, and worthy of our esteem, care, and *caring*?

The Need to Be Seen

This image, inspired by the work of Dutch graphic artist Maurits Cornelis Escher, captures the essence of this delicate interaction (see Figure 2.1). It could very well have been entitled *Dignity in the Eye of the Beholder*,[3] given that healthcare providers bear witness to, and hence are the *beholders* of, their patients' experiences. Notice that the image reflected in the eye of the beholder is that of an elderly woman. Whatever else we might assume about her, we know she has a home; surroundings that are familiar to her; possessions including books, photographs, and paintings indicative of interests, values, and a history that is entirely independent of whatever healthcare ailments she happens to have. The ability to provide this kind of holistic, all-encompassing reflection is entirely dependent on the attitude of the healthcare provider and is key to preserving patient dignity.

In each encounter patients look toward us for recognition and affirmation. When we only see their ailment and how that condition might behave

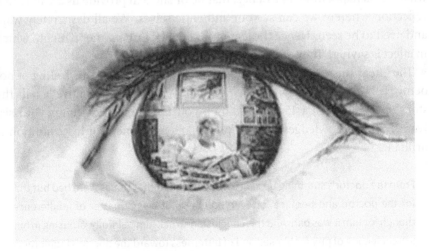

Figure 2.1 Dignity in the eye of the beholder.

therapeutically, patients are apt to feel personhood has been sacrificed. *Do you understand me? Do you know what I am going through? Do you know there is more to me than can be captured in my medical chart?* Metaphorically patients are looking for an affirming reflection in the eye of the beholder. The absence of such a reflection will leave them feeling that they no longer really exist, at least not those parts that cannot be expressed in terms of symptoms, laboratory tests, or objective clinical findings. If the only thing they see in the eye of the beholder is their illness, a differential diagnosis, and problem checklist, they will be left feeling that they are nothing more than their illness. But when they recognize themselves reflected in the eye of the healthcare provider, dignity and personhood are most likely to be upheld. This echoes Arthur Schopenhauer's notion of dignity being dependent on the opinion of others regarding our worth and our fear of that opinion.[4] When healthcare providers offer patients a reflection wherein they can see themselves and the entirety of who they are, a reflection they need not fear, they are likely to feel that dignity is being upheld and that patienthood has not eclipsed personhood.

Reflect on a personal healthcare experience. Recall not only the presenting problem or concern that drew you into care, but the feelings of vulnerability, uncertainty, or fear that likely accompanied you into that office, clinic, or hospital. You probably remember at some point hoping that you placed your trust in capable hands. While you may or may not remember all the details of what took place or all that was said, you will no doubt remember how you were made to feel. We enter these encounters with the wish to be understood, hoping the healthcare provider will see and appreciate us in the context of whatever is happening; in essence, that he or she will provide us an affirming reflection wherein we can see our authentic selves. We all desperately want and need to be seen. Hence the lament, "I felt like just another patient," which in effect is saying, "they didn't really see me."

The Great Russian writer Leo Tolstoy perfectly captures this feeling of not being seen in his masterpiece *The Death of Ivan Ilyich*.[5] This novella tells the story of the death of a 45-year-old high-court judge in 19th-century Russia. Ivan Ilyich acknowledges that his physician's assessment of his condition is brilliant.

> From the doctor's summing up Ivan Ilyich concluded that things were bad but that for the doctor, and perhaps for everybody else, it was a matter of indifference, though for him it was bad. And this conclusion struck him painfully, arousing in him a great feeling of pity for himself and of bitterness toward the doctor's indifference to a matter of such importance.

Ivan Ilyich desperately needed to be seen, which is something his doctor failed to appreciate or offer.

Attitude and Mindfulness

Being mindful that attitude shapes healthcare encounters is more complex than it might first appear. Everyone entering healthcare has been socialized in a particular fashion. Like anyone else, who you are has been shaped by the way you were raised; by the culture, values, and beliefs you've been exposed to; and by the biases and prejudices that surround you. Collectively these influences contribute to what you sense is good and bad, what is right and wrong, what is valuable and what is not, what is sacred and what is dispensable. If patients are looking for a reflection of themselves in your eye, these influences determine the contours of the lens within which those reflections will be shaped.

Attitude describes the internalized filters through which we see the world and, of course, determines how we see our patients. These filters usually operate outside of conscious awareness. They shape our assumptions and worldviews, creating mindsets that feel intuitive, immutable, and, fundamentally, are experienced as part of who we are. Asking someone to describe these filters is like asking a person born color-blind to explain their visual experience. The response is likely to be, "it feels perfectly normal," or they don't tend to give it much thought. If this is the only reality they have known, there is no basis for comparison. While they may deem their visual perception to be accurate, it is, nonetheless, distorted and inconsistent with how others see or experience the world. Asking them to reflect on their perceptions, however, indicates that others can appreciate shades of color beyond the spectrum of black and white. Posing the question makes them mindful that their perception is idiosyncratic and not universally held. Being human means being confined within a unique set of realities that shape who we are and how we intuitively experience and see the world around us. It takes mindfulness, a reminder that we are seeing the world through invisible filters, to put us in touch with these imperceptible and formidable influences. Without questioning our assumptions and raising them into consciousness, it is easy to be led astray.

My sister, Ellen Chochinov, was born with cerebral palsy. To say this affected her is a gross understatement. It was part of who she was and certainly presented physical and emotional challenges every day of her life. But cerebral palsy was not the entirety of my sister's existence. Although medicine has found ways to explain and categorize the specifics of cerebral palsy, as Catherine Frazee points out, "this no more describes [the] experience of disability than does the medical description of puberty describe what it means to be 13 years old."[6] While some people might assume that Ellen's extensive disabilities meant her life consisted of little more than suffering, on a dance floor, given her less than stellar driving skills, the only people who suffered were those whose toes she crushed under the mighty weight of her electric wheelchair.

Several years before she died at the age of 55, she was admitted to hospital, this time because of acute respiratory symptoms that quickly led to a transfer to intensive care. Cerebral palsy expresses itself in a variety of ways depending on the degree of anoxic insult the brain suffers at the time of birth. Complications can include spinal deformities, muscle wasting, atrophy, spasticity, and chronic pain, to name but a few, all of which Ellen could claim were part of her body's unique and complex repertoire. The current respiratory episode was one of many, albeit the most serious to date. Perhaps severe kyphosis had compromised the size of her pleural cavity, or maybe her diaphragm, as most every other part of her body, was underperforming. Respiratory capacity had never been her strong suit. I never recall Ellen being able to blow out a single candle on her birthday cake, not even if her life depended on it. That did not curtail her enjoyment of being celebrated; she loved being the center of attention. She loved time at the lake with our family, she loved her friends, watching movies, particularly romances or ones whose plot involved people living with adversity. In Chochinov vernacular, such entertainment was rated *E* for Ellen. She enjoyed traveling to the extent this was possible; good food, especially things my mother cooked or my father did up on the barbeque; sweet desserts and chocolate milk.

Those of us who knew Ellen well understood that her life was complex, and while her body may have been severely misshapen, twisted, and distorted, that did not preclude her capacity to love or to be loved. That day in intensive care, between her oxygen mask and increasing levels of somnolence due to breathing difficulties, she was no longer able to speak for herself. It was becoming increasingly apparent to everyone, her family and healthcare providers alike, that she was deteriorating, and we were entering into previously uncharted territory. As we began to teeter dangerously close to a decision about whether she would need to be intubated, the attending intensivist approached me with a cryptic and chilling question: "Does she read magazines?" I had worked as a consultant on this unit many times. I was familiar with the clinical milieu, with the language, the messages, and metamessages. What I was not familiar with was being on the other side of the provider–patient equation. "Does she read magazines" seems like an innocent question, but its subtext is profound and a question whose answer I knew could tip the scale precariously hovering between life and death. The subtext read as follows: "she looks and is twisted like a pretzel, and you know we don't intubate pretzels." Realizing the gravity of his question and the implications I knew would be attached to my response hit me with a wave of nausea. After a moment's pause and reflection, I responded, "Yes, she reads magazines, but only when she is between novels."[7]

Attitude and Perception

To be clear, the clinicians looking after Ellen that day were not bad people. In fact the intensive care they provided was impeccable, and, mercifully, with superb supportive measures, she managed to recover without being intubated. However, there is no doubt that they saw Ellen in a particular way, based on their own life experience and having absorbed a lifetime of messages, biases, and assumptions regarding what it means to be disabled. Popular culture and the global media are constantly exposing us to images of the idealized perfect body (young, thin, and toned) and story lines that privilege autonomy, power, and wealth. Continuous exposure to these messages fashions attitudes, no less than exposure to contaminated air determines health and our ability to breathe. No one is immune from these influences, including the people who worked in ICU that day. Attitudes are the internalized filters through which we see our patients. That day, her ICU physician saw a woman whose body was shaped like a pretzel through the eyes of someone who was able-bodied, middle-aged, Caucasian, and male. That is not an accusation, condemnation, or verdict; rather, it is a simple statement of fact.

In the moment, he was likely as unaware of the complex determinants of his judgment—that perhaps not being too aggressive was best, given the circumstances—as we were regarding why her respiratory status had suddenly declined. No doubt he was attempting to respond from a position of beneficence. Given the opportunity to explain his motivation, he would likely have shared his concern about what he perceived to be her suffering, the futility of being overly aggressive, and the wisdom of letting nature take its course. But perceptions are just that. They are an interpretation of circumstances based on an appreciation of what we can observe and recognize. Perceptions will always be shaped according to those filters through which we bear witness. Even compassion, which requires an awareness of the suffering of another and the wish to respond to it, depends on perception. If how we appreciate suffering is shaped by filters that can distort our perception, a genuine, even well-motivated attempt to respond compassionately might result in care that is entirely discordant with the patient's wishes and values (see "Distorted Compassion," Chapter 3).

Dr. Bruce Martin has been a family physician for nearly 45 years, including extensive experience working in Canada's remote Arctic. His skills, wisdom, and caring are nothing less than extraordinary. He describes how attitude and perception sometimes results in criticism:

> by my southern and urban colleagues that northern patients don't commit enough to their own care. They'll cite instances when the patient was supposed to come down for a colposcopy and never did and now, she has metastatic carcinoma of the cervix. To which I say perhaps I have an understanding of why she didn't come. She has a husband who's the hunter gatherer for all intents and purposes, and she has been asked to come down in the peak of his harvesting season. They live in the Artic, and she's got four kids to look after and culturally she's looking after her parents, too. So that's why she didn't come down. It wasn't because she doesn't care, it wasn't because she doesn't look after her own health, it is just the context of the community, the culture and the context of her own life that would make coming difficult. Besides you didn't give her much notice. If you gave her another week's notice for the appointment instead of the night before, perhaps she could have made arrangements with her sister to look after them and perhaps I wouldn't now be looking after the unbelievable consequences of her metastatic disease at the age of 25 with four kids. So again, having an understanding of the individual, the family, the culture and the community helps me to promote a better approach to care and a better understanding for patients, rather than passing judgement based on too little information and unjustified assumptions.

Attitude and Being a Good Person

Anyone working in healthcare having patient contact must remember that their attitude toward patients and families will invariably and indelibly influence the healthcare experience. The complexities of those attitudes require constant scrutiny and attention, given they are shaped by influences beyond conscious awareness. Dr. Mike Harlos is a nationally lauded, retired palliative care physician and most trusted colleague. He believes that being a good doctor means having a solid medical knowledge base, having technical skills, and being a good person, which includes knowing yourself. He is among the finest physicians I have ever worked with and embodies those ingredients in spades. Aside from superb technical abilities and knowledge, he is quick to point out that, "you can't address suffering without connecting with the nonphysical elements of who that person is." Which is why, whenever he teaches medical residents about communication skills and decision-making, he asks them to consider, "'What would a good person do in this situation?' And this doesn't just have to be your patient, just do it with every person, with the waiter, the guy who cut you off in traffic, with everyone. This is a kind of attentiveness to the needs of others."

Dr. Harlos says that being a good person requires a degree of self-awareness that continuously informs your attitude. "For instance, struggling out of a grocery store with an armful of groceries, a few steps behind someone in front of you. Some people allow the door to close in your face behind them as they walk through, not even checking to see if it might need to be held open for someone. Others check behind them, hold the door, and might even offer help carrying the groceries." He says that it is very likely "that people who take that extra moment to help are continuously vigilant. *What would a good person do? What would I want if that were me?*" He points out, however, that "being a good person is no more a one-time decision than deciding to lose 30 pounds. You can't just decide it. You have to live it. You have to be mindful every time you have the option to take a set of stairs or not or eat that desert or take a pass." He shared a conversation he had with a religious friend who told him that living according to Orthodox Jewish traditions and precepts requires mindfulness, "like a thread of consciousness that becomes woven into the fabric of our being."

Mindfulness, humility, and being a good person go hand in hand. Good and mindful people recognize that their own perceptions and judgments bear scrutiny, that they are fallible, limited, and may sometimes miss the mark. Humility sees us concede that our perceptions may be imperfect, insisting that we consider alternative explanations for where our assumptions might initially take us.

Attitude and Prejudice

There is a razor thin line between the notion of pre-judgment and prejudice. The Latin derivative for prejudice, *prae judicium*, means *previous judgment*, *damage*, or *opinion formed in advance*. There is no doubt that pre-judgment or opinions formed in advance, that is formed before knowing or appreciating something sufficiently, can inflict great harm and do irreparable damage. Dr. Michael Moffatt is a wise and experienced retired pediatrician with a life-long passion for northern and aboriginal health issues. During his practice, it was not uncommon for him to have critically ill children flown into Winnipeg for more intensive monitoring and treatment. On one such occasion he recalled admitting a First Nations 2-year-old little girl with bronchiolitis from a small remote community in northern Manitoba. Within a few days of her arrival, the nursing staff had become increasingly concerned that her mother was not visiting regularly and, in their opinion, was not spending sufficient time with her sick child. Without knowing what to make of it, concern shifted to innuendo and innuendo to accusations, wherein they judged her to be *uncaring and a bad mother*.

By way of damage control, Dr. Moffatt sought to defuse the situation by trying to find out why this young mother was so disturbingly absent. Her explanation was heartbreaking. She had come into the city prior to her daughter's admission to look after her now hospitalized, dying mother. Her 6-year-old daughter had traveled with her, given there was no one at home to leave her with. Mother and daughter were now staying in a small hotel room, isolated, away from friends and family, with little money and virtually no support. Her days consisted of tending to her older daughter; whenever she could, taking a bus to spend time with her dying mother and then making her way across the city to see her younger, hospitalized, daughter. The initial pre-judgments, while perhaps coming from a place of concern, could hardly have been further off the mark and led to alienation, resentment, and distrust.

Sue Bates, the former Director of Patient Navigation at CancerCare Manitoba, told a similar story of false assumptions and prejudice.

This was a pediatric case of a 2-year-old with rhabdomyosarcoma. The course of treatment prescribed was long and hard, starting with radiation therapy along with chemotherapy for nearly a year. The mother was a First Nations woman about 25 years old, with two other children, one a baby and the other a 5-year-old son with mild cerebral palsy. Her partner had gone back to the reserve, so she was told by the physician that "you're on your own and you're not going to cope unless you give up school." She had been funded for school by the band, since she was bright and articulate and getting top marks, and yet she was being encouraged to *put your child in care*. That's probably not the best approach, especially given the history of the Residential Schools in Canada. She fought all the way, but the whole relationship with that family broke down during the entire time of that care. There was once she actually failed to bring her child in for treatment; it turned out that she and her grandma both had a really bad gastro bug and the child needed to come in for radiation. They threatened her on the phone with Child and Family Services. That was totally undignified and showed a lack of respect. They weren't saying they were never coming again, just that they were sick and can't bring him this time. There were a couple of times that she herself was sick and admitted to hospital, and she would have the doctors and nurses ring us up because she was so scared of what we'd do because she couldn't get her son into us. She'd have her brother bring him or use any family members she could to get through that. But she managed to stick with the treatment plan and didn't give up school.

Attitude and the Platinum Rule

Some healthcare providers feel that so long as their outlook toward patients and families includes the Golden Rule, *do unto others as you would have them do unto you*, they will not go too far astray. Within medicine, this means treating patients and families the way we would want to be treated or would want our loved ones to be treated under similar circumstances. There is deep wisdom in this aphorism, some form of which can be found within many religions and ethical traditions. The Golden Rule is based on the idea of reciprocity and our being able to see ourselves in others. "If I were that patient, how would I want to be treated? What if this was my mother, my father, sister, or brother? How would I want them to be treated?" Dr. Michael West knows and lives this mantra. He is an exceptional neurosurgeon who graduated from medicine in 1973, then completed a neurosurgery residency and a PhD in physiology. He pioneered gamma knife surgery in Canada and is a strong proponent of technology that has virtually transformed his field. He says, "When I speak with people, I've often had a picture in mind; if this was a relative or myself, how would I want to be treated?" No doubt, the ability to project ourselves into our patients' experiences offers a profound and humanizing perspective.

Failure to adhere to the Golden Rule can have dire consequences for patients and families as well as healthcare providers. Dr. Harlos recalls being contacted by a community nurse, taking care of an oncology patient who was palliative, but not registered on the palliative care program.

> The patient had died at about 2 o'clock in the morning and none of the preparation as far as all the proper paperwork needed for an anticipated home death had been done. The nurse called the oncologist and he just proceeded to absolutely ream her out: "How dare you. The person is dead. There is no medical emergency to justify you waking me up. The family can wait until tomorrow morning when I start working, so sit tight." The family had to wait with a corpse in the room, which they found very disturbing and the nurse was upset.

Clearly this physician did not stop to consider how he would have wanted to be treated if he were in this situation. In a similar vein of failing to adhere to the Golden Rule, Dr. Harlos recalls filling in forms because the involved physician didn't want to waste time filling them in.

> These forms are often to indicate that this person is expected to die at home, which means the family doesn't have to call 911, police, or the coroner. There are several physicians in town who think it's beneath them, they won't do it because they don't get paid for it. Yet it takes me 1 minute to do and they won't do it, so they expect if the family calls 911, that resuscitation will be attempted on this patient and that's it. If this was your mom, would you still think that would be okay?

The Golden Rule, however, has its limitations in that it requires there be some alignment or overlap between how we see ourselves and how we see others. So long as patients' values and priorities align with our own, we can readily anticipate their needs based on how we would want to be treated in a similar situation. We might even just assume that their priorities align with our own since ours strike us as so reasonable. The further our worldview and circumstances deviate from that of our patients, the more likely the Golden Rule falls short of meeting their needs and expectations. Our own biases and perceptions of current and anticipated future suffering can lead to decisions and recommendations discordant with patients' perceptions, values, and goals of care. A *Platinum Rule*, particularly in these circumstances, might provide a worthy alternative: *Do unto patients as they would want done unto themselves.* This implicates not only clinical decisions but treating (that is, acting toward) patients as they would want to be treated. This means knowing who patients are as persons, hence guiding treatment decisions, as well as shaping a tone of care based on genuine compassion and respect. When stated preferences are less than certain, it is important to explore their and their family's values informing treatment recommendations. Not all patient preferences can or should be accommodated, especially when they are driven by nihilistic self-loathing ("I don't want anything") or motivated by expectations that exceed any objective reality ("I want everything"). Even in those instances, it is important to understand what patients want and why. While patients' choices may or may not align with our own values or priorities, a platinum standard acknowledges that we cannot always be the perfect, infallible barometer of our patients' wants and needs. For example, when Dr. Harlos would tell substitute decision makers,

> the question isn't what you want us to do, for example treating their father's pneumonia, but asking what that person would want done. "Imagine your dad 6 months

ago and tell me what he would want us to do. Let's imagine sitting with him at his own bedside and imagine 'okay, dad, you've been in hospital for 2 weeks. You've been unconscious for 2 days. The doctor says he doesn't think you are going to make it through the night, but he also thinks you have pneumonia, which in theory is treatable, but nobody knows how you're going to respond to that. They can keep you comfortable with or without treatment. What would your dad say?" And 90% of the time the person says my dad would say "leave me alone." Or they say in fact my dad a week ago said "I wish I could just go to sleep and not wake up again." The question is not what you would want done, but what, in this instance, your father would want done *unto himself*.

Dr. Harlos shared another case where a person was dying on the ward.

He was married, had a very good relationship with his wife who was his healthcare proxy, and was Jewish but didn't follow it in an orthodox way. His brother, who was from out of town, was very, very orthodox. The patient's healthcare directive said "I don't want IV fluids when I'm dying, just leave me be." His brother came to be with him as he was dying and said, "I can't support this. It's not part of what I understand the orthodox approach to end of life." He said to the wife, "if this is the approach taken (no IV fluids), we're done. I don't think I can be a part of your family any more." So I said to the wife that the spirit of the healthcare directive was not to prolong his dying. Again, I said, "let's imagine your husband like he was 6 months ago, let's sit him down and talk this out. What do you think he would say, knowing the impact and what's at stake in this situation?" And she said he would say "give me some IV fluids, since it's not expected to prolong things and isn't much of a burden." Again, the decision-making rested not on what the wife wanted done, but rather on *what her husband would have wanted done* in this particular instance.

Dr. Harlos recalled another case of a woman dying in the emergency ward of metastatic lung cancer.

When I went down there, she was unresponsive, with irregular breathing, thready pulse, mottled, looking like she would die in the next several hours. She had two daughters. One said, "my best friend died recently and they just kept plugging away and trying to stop it, it went on for weeks. I don't want this dragged on for mom—I want you to just take out that intravenous and don't do any antibiotics and just keep her comfortable." The other daughter said, "I can't give up on mom. I know she's dying. I don't want CPR but if you guys do nothing, we're done as a family."

So, I said to the first daughter, "you know your mom already has the IV in, so simply leaving it in place would not add to her suffering. And the antibiotics that are ordered will not stop her from dying—her condition is far too advanced and overwhelming to be improved with antibiotics. So, I can assure you that by continuing what's being done, she will not have her suffering prolonged. But can we imagine what your mom would say trying to reconcile this difficult situation. I kind of think most moms would say, okay, given me the antibiotics if it means that my two daughters are going to still talk to each other."

So I kept the antibiotics, kept the IV, she got one more dose at 2 in the morning and died at 5 later that morning.

The daughter was asked, in essence, to invoke a platinum standard. "How would your mother, not you, have wanted this situation dealt with?"

Maria Fraser is a remarkable nurse manager whose practice has taken her around the world, including more than 20 years in Canada's far north. She thinks that to meet the needs of patients, one must "understand and respect their culture and beliefs, including their spirituality, and not have expectations that they know and feel what I believe in. Then you can provide them care that they will feel comfortable with"—in other words, the Platinum Rule, treat them as *they* would want us to treat them. In reflecting on spiritual care, Maria recalled a drowning accident. "The whole health center was just screaming and wailing. We were trying to resuscitate this child. But the moment the doctor said, "would you like the minister to come and pray?" there was dead silence. They appreciated the doctor for suggesting that. It had a calming effect on them, and they appreciated the fact that he looked into what they believe to be of use to them."

From Maria's viewpoint, knowing how to treat clients means appreciating their personal circumstances and arriving at solutions that acknowledge and reflect their perspectives. "I worked in the reserves way out in the bushes. Most of those client's didn't have the basic necessities of life. I couldn't tell them to go home and feed your little child chicken noodle soup. But if I said, "you go and get some chickens. . . ." I knew they had chickens. I knew they had to slaughter the chicken and boil the meat and bones, so I help them utilize what they had and not suggest something that was beyond their reach. In my work with the Inuit people, I try to understand and ask them lots of questions and make them feel comfortable and ask them, "What do you think is best for you?" They come up with a suggestion, and I make some, and I ask them for their feedback. For instance, a child comes to you with a fever: "So how do you think you are going to get that fever down?" It takes a lot of time, but if I tell her to go and give Tylenol and if she doesn't have

Tylenol, then it is futile. So I ask her, "How do you think or what do you have to get this fever down?" If she says I can give her a drink or a cold bath, I'll say, "yes that is fine." But if I say give her a cool bath and she doesn't have water, then that doesn't work. So, I try to ask questions about what they would like done and what do they envision would be best for them. And I want to respect their views first. Value their judgment and what they have to say. Show respect for their values rather than forcing my southern way of thinking.

> They eat a lot of whale blubber, seal meat with a very high content of fat in it. And if that is the sole diet, then it is going to cause gallstones and gastroesophageal reflux. But that is their way, that is their food. So, if you tell them to change that, it has to be done in a way that they do it in moderation and supplement it with other foods that are affordable and food that they can get that is not so high in fat. So, they might be told, "when the time was cold, because you ate blubber, that is why you are sick. Because you ate seal meat, that is why you are sick. Because you ate raw meat, that is why you got a stomach infection or gastroenteritis." The middle-aged and older people eat the traditional food like frozen meat, frozen fish, uncooked, so it is very upsetting to them to say "that has caused you to be sick." I think it is the approach of how you say it, so they don't feel that their staple food is going to cause illness.

The Platinum Rule requires deep appreciation and respect for the perspective of the patient, family, and their community and a willingness to learn about that perspective. Twenty years of working on the Arctic Circle has given Maria a sense of awe and even reverence for the Inuit culture and ways, including the tenacity and strength it takes to survive this harsh environment. In reflecting on this, she told the following story:

> A man and his wife were traveling by land on a snowmobile with a sled attached to it and on the sled was all their camping gear, their food, and some caribou skins. This was their mode of travel, and they would travel from one community to another, which would be 6 or 7 hours. But accidents do happen. This couple hit thin ice and went down into the water and got hypothermic. The husband remarkably didn't give up. His wife was on the sled, and he was on the skidoo. As the skidoo was going down, the skis got caught on the ice flow and he managed to grab and jump onto that patch of ice. She was right in the middle of the water when they went down and she was struggling, but she took that caribou skin and she stayed afloat by holding onto this skin. Eventually the husband managed to pull her out of the water and put her onto the land and she was shivering.

What I have learned from the people here that has remained with me is that they have a tremendous sense of being practical on how to do things to get out of a situation like that. I would have been so scared. But what I leaned from them is that they held onto every ounce of energy they had to save themselves and try every possible means to come out of that water. Yes, they were scared but somehow their fight to get onto that land meant that they had a very strong sense of survival.

Without respect and understanding of this cultural perspective and adherence to the Platinum Rule, it is simply not possible to provide care that will resonate with the patient's values and goals of care.

B Stands for Behavior

A core precept of cognitive behavioral therapy is that how we think has a direct bearing on how we feel, which in turn influences how we behave. Attitude denotes how we see and shapes how we feel about our patients. Attitude is the lens through which we see the world, including our patients and their families, and is ingrained into who we are as people. As much as what we say or do not say, or what we do or do not do, our attitude enters into every clinical encounter. More so than anything else about us as healthcare professionals, attitude mediates our ability to provide patients *caring* and opens the doorway to trust. While attitude is internally held, *behavior* is the outward manifestation of a dignity-conserving attitude. These behaviors are observable, are experienced by others, and constitute the essence of dignity-conserving practices. They demonstrate our ability to see and appreciate patients as persons. Conversely, failure to truly see our patients and their families has observable behavioral manifestations that can undermine or taint our efforts to provide dignity-conserving care (Table 2.1).

Table 2.1 Dignity-conserving behaviors

Ways of seeing the patient	Failure to see the patient
Maintaining patient contact	Avoiding patient contact/Abandonment
Being completely present	Partial presence (e.g., distractions) or absence
Making eye contact, sitting	Averting eye contact, standing
Individualizing engagement	Making engagements generic (e.g., elderspeak)

Maintaining Patient Contact

Knowing that attitude mediates patient experience should lead to the realization that *presence, being with the patient,* has profound clinical and therapeutic import. Conversely, not showing up or abandonmesent is the epitome of *failure to see* the patient. Patient contact is typically associated with designated, time-specific tasks and things that have objective and measurable utility. Providing medication, registering a patient at triage, taking a history, providing postsurgical instructions, obtaining vital signs; each of these might appear in a job description, require certain competencies, and can be signed off on a medical chart or checklist. Like countless such tasks, each falls within the domain of *doing to* patients. They are usually action-oriented, can be documented, and, once executed, can be set aside as complete. With a dignity-conserving attitude comes behavior that affirms that *being with a patient,* in its own right, can be as critical and healing as *doing to a patient.* Hence the sage adage, *don't just do something, stand there!*

Being with is not a singular event but a process that continuously evolves throughout the course of caring for patients and families. *Being with* does not typically appear in a chart, nor will the skills and sensibilities required to do *being with* well appear in a job description or healthcare professional training curriculum. Yet dignity in care requires that we show up and that we understand that our commitment to do so, no matter what the circumstances, is vital and non-negotiable. Dr. Mike West says, "the technology has improved what we can do for patients; it has converted some inoperable tumors into tumors that can be resected; vascular malformations that couldn't be treated before and could take the patient's life, can now be treated with gamma knife in a day procedure. But between all of the tools, monitors and scopes," he says, "you have to look and remind yourself that the patient is still there. When technology reaches its limitations to help the patient, some surgeons just can't handle that. They get to the point where they can't do something for the patient and the patient ends up being deserted. They just don't know what to do anymore. It's not that they're not interested, but they can't handle it. I've seen this happen with medical and surgical care. Eventually they stop returning the patient's calls because they don't know what to say. They don't know how to deal with them. They don't want to bring them in and be frank about what's happening. That's left for somebody else; *it's not my problem.*"

"With increasing technology", says Dr. West, "there's a tendency to transfer some of those communication responsibilities to other people, such as the nurse or the physician assistant. Physicians try to convince themselves that they are so important that they need to be in the operating room, or be in the clinic, or administering chemotherapy; that their time is so important that they have to do those very technical things rather than sitting down and talking to the patient. They might spend 4 or 5 hours in surgery, sometimes even more, and yet they consider sitting down with someone for 20 or 30 minutes too long." Dr. West recognizes that "it is so easy to fall into that trap." He will purposefully "slow down so the person does not feel like they're being rushed. So often," he says, "I hear from patients that they saw a physician who was supposed to be good, but they didn't get a chance to ask any questions. So, I think that a sign of respect for the patient and for the family is giving them the opportunity to speak. To let you know what troubles them without interruption. To listen to them and let them ask their questions." Despite being an extremely busy neurosurgeon, his approach is to "let patients and families ask questions until they have nothing left to ask, and then suggest that they can contact you again if they think of anything further. As you get more experienced, you get more complicated referrals. You're dealing with life and death, function and loss of function. Sometimes they've heard that they might not wake up or they might wake up paralyzed. It's an extraordinary trust that they place in a surgeon. You should sit with that patient and family until their questions are exhausted. Considering that we spend 4, 5, 8 hours in surgery, sitting down with someone for 20 or 30 minutes isn't too long or too much to ask."

Healthcare providers and healthcare systems are geared to fix things, and the further away patients move from a *fix it* paradigm, the more regular contact can start to wane. This can happen when a treatment or course of treatment is completed or when curative options start to run out. That is usually when the most dreaded words in all of medicine are uttered, "there is nothing more we can do for you," words that should be expunged from our medical vocabulary. Dr. West says that, all too often, patients and families find themselves abandoned in their time of most dire need. "I do find that it is more common that residents in surgery are most interested in the techniques of surgery and don't really pay as much attention to the pre- and postoperative care. In their minds, that is not what they are there for, although the best residents will have a real acknowledgment about the holistic approach to patients." He recalled the case of a gentleman with a craniopharyngioma.

These are complex cases because they involve endocrine complications. This patient had surgery, and they couldn't do very much about the tumor. His hypothalamus was damaged, so there were difficulties with consciousness, fluid balance, temperature regulation, blood pressure regulation, and all of those homeostatic mechanisms. The attending physician, who would know more about the management of these complications, was just not involved in the postoperative care. You could see one complication after another occurring because of the inexperience of the people who were left behind to deal with the fluid balance, temperature regulation, blood pressure, and supplementation of the pituitary hormones. The patient was in a coma one day because nobody had ordered any replacement steroids for steroid supplementation.

I was asked to see the patient as a second opinion, and my first inclination was to talk to the physician and say, "What is happening? Here is this family and they want to talk to me because this patient had surgery 2 months ago and you have seen him and the family once." I think part of it is the intimidation of having to face failure and having to discuss this with the patient and with the family. I think to some degree that is because of how terrible it is talking to somebody when something that we've done hasn't worked out as expected. Of course, if you have carefully prepared and discussed all of this with the patient and the family, then they know all the possibilities. But still, you have failed to accomplish what you have set out to do. So it is extra challenging to walk into that room and talk to them and explain issues and deal with complications that occur because the patient isn't well. But when you work past that, it is rare that there is any ill will if you have shown a continued interest and involvement in the patient's welfare. I think they just respect and appreciate the fact that you are still on board. In the Hippocratic tradition, cure sometimes, treat often, and comfort always.

A commitment to nonabandonment extends not only to patients but to their families as well. Dr. West recalled a young lady with a young family who just out of the blue came in with an acute collapse from a ruptured aneurysm with lots of blood in and around the brain.

All of the predictors were that things were not going to go well. She had hydrocephalus that required a drain and the amount of blood suggested that she was going to develop vasospasm, which leads to a high risk of having a stroke. This is the worst kind of scenario in medicine. A young patient with a young family who you know, from the start, is not going to do well. People tend to back off a little because they don't want to get involved, and they know that things are going to go badly. In that circumstance I felt that it was important to lay that picture out up front. We spent a lot of time talking to them about what the issues were and the potential complications. While I said we were going to be very aggressive and had all the technology that we needed, they needed to understand that a lot of damage had already been done. And she did develop complications. At that point it is not so much about surgery but more of an ICU issue. So the surgeons had to back off at that point, despite the fact that we were the first connection, with intimate knowledge about the patient and her family. You then have a sequence of caregivers who are there for a day at a time. They don't know the family and they don't know the previous discussions.

I made sure to continue following the patient, even though the care had gone beyond where I had to be there to manage the blood pressure, the respirator, and those sorts of things. But I would go look out for the family and make sure to talk to them about the progress and the prognosis and how it was becoming clearer that this wouldn't end well. I talked with them and prepared them by saying, "if at this point she survives, she would have very serious deficits," and describe those deficits and prepared them for that last conversation, saying that "we know that she can't recover from this, so we need to look at stopping the treatment and maybe salvage something meaningful by organ donation." My motivation in staying involved is not to make it easier for me. The easiest thing for a surgeon to say is, "I'm not needed here and I'm just not going to follow the patient anymore." But staying involved is all about compassion and empathy. You get involved, you are almost becoming part of that family. You can almost see yourself in their position. You are looking back and you are seeing your own family, and thinking, "I can't walk away from this because I would want somebody to do this if I was in that position." It becomes a subconscious thing as to how I would want somebody to deal with me if I was that person with three kids and my wife was on a respirator. I think I stay involved by putting myself in the position of the patient. It's very emotional. As I'm going into the family room with a resident I say, "this may take 10 minutes or half an hour, but I think we have to let the family ask every question, make every accusation, question every step along the way without taking any offense to it." If you are talking about end-of-life or end-of-management discussions, you have to let them ask all of the questions that they can. In these situations, I tell residents, "a half hour with these patients and families can be as taxing and challenging as 5 hours in the OR." It is very stressful because you aren't sure how they are going to react, and you are the person who has failed to get them through this. It is hardly a time when people can be grateful. They will have lots of questions. And if they want to have other family members there, let them. I think we need to be sincere and show interest, and I think we do that by showing up and letting them ask their questions."

Being Completely Present

A vital element of patient contact is being sure that when you arrive, you show up *completely*. There are so many things that can interfere with seeing our patients, and only partially arriving at their bedside is one of them. Distractions in the healthcare are everywhere. Not even a closed examination room or hospital room door ensures complete insulation from outside interferences. While many of these intrusions are normal and seemingly inescapable, left unchecked, they can thwart *showing up completely* and undermine our ability to respond to patients and their families in the most effective manner possible.

The most portable intrusions we take into patient encounters are those inside of our heads. They are the various personal and professional worries, preoccupations, and distractions that follow us wherever we go. All of us live complex lives, and the way we conduct ourselves in clinical settings is vulnerable to being shaped by everything and anything that might be on our mind, things that should ideally remain outside of the therapeutic moment. Perhaps there are personal issues we are carrying from the home front, family conflicts or obligations that need to be addressed or worked through, financial demands or pressures that should be dealt with, personal health issues that ought to be attended to. Similarly, there may be myriad professional issues that can be difficult to compartmentalize; administrative demands, teaching obligations, collegial relationships that need to be managed; academic challenges; and, perhaps most prominent of all, daily pressures to fulfill our clinical obligations for patients and families. Depending on what is going on in our heads and in our hearts, separating those distractions from the job at hand can be difficult to manage. Doing so, however, by way of compartmentalizing whatever is competing for our attention and being fully present, attentive, and curious, ensures optimal therapeutic communication (see Chapter 3).

Technology is constantly challenging our ability to negotiate this separation. Handheld devices, such as smartphones, pagers, and the like connect each of us to the entire world, even when we are seemingly alone with our patients. In regular social discourse these devices and an ethos of always being in touch and constant multitasking are increasingly becoming the norm. However, in healthcare, the context is different or certainly ought to be. Patients are more fragile and vulnerable and having a distracted healthcare provider can easily be interpreted as *something or someone else is more important than I am. You are not listening to me. I guess I don't deserve your full and complete attention.* A medical resident shared his recollection of being on call with a physician who turned out to be an *inattentive* attending. As is typical for ward rounds, the medical staff and trainees crowded into the patient's room with the resident taking charge of presenting the case and highlighting the various salient medical facts and findings. The medical students flanked both sides of the patient's bed, while the resident stood more closely by the patient's side. The attending settled into a chair placed behind this throng of learners, making himself comfortable next to a small table strewn with magazines and newspapers. As the resident proceeded to describe the case, he noticed that his attending was seemingly distracted by an apparently all too tempting array of reading material. Despite the patient's efforts to convince himself otherwise, any pretense of being listened to dissolved with the undeniable sound of rustling newsprint and the flipping of pages.

Showing up to see patients counts for a great deal, but how you behave and hold yourself once you arrive is also critically important. Before saying a word, posture and body language convey critical messages that, given patients' exquisite sensitivity, will be held up to scrutiny. Do you, for example, stand over the patient at their bedside, or pull up a chair where you can see them on an equal plane, eye to eye? The act of sitting transmits an important message. Besides alleviating a perceived power differential patients might feel with someone towering over them, sitting conveys the intent to take some time. Patients perceive the amount of time their healthcare provider spends with them as longer when the healthcare provider sits rather than stands. In an intriguing study by a group of researchers from the University of Kansas, this hypothesis was cleverly put to the test.[8] These investigators, affiliated with the Department of Nursing and the Department of Neurosurgery, designed a randomized trial that recruited 120 post-elective spinal surgery patients. Patients were randomly assigned a *standing* or *sitting* follow-up visit with their surgeon. The actual length of each visit was timed and compared afterward with the patient's perception of their visit.

In all instances patients perceived the length of the follow-up visit as much longer than the actual timed duration of the visit. In instances when the physician stood, patients felt their 1 minute, 28 second visit had lasted almost three times longer. When the physician sat, the perceptual distortion was nearly fivefold greater. The study investigators also reported that sitting not only changed time perceptions, but also the degree of satisfaction patients reported within those encounters. Specifically, 95% of comments from patients who had received a *seated visit* were positive, such as "the doctor took the time to sit and listen," and "he sat down long enough to get all of my questions answered." Overall, 95% of these patients expressed satisfaction with the encounter. They felt their questions were well addressed and expressed a better understanding of their condition. On the other hand, only 61% of comments from patients who had a *standing visit* were positive, with various negative comments to the effect that "I didn't have time to ask the doctor any questions," and "he was in and out of my room before I even knew what was going on."

Finding tangible ways of letting patients know that we are prepared to listen to them and spend time with them is clearly important, and sitting conveys those messages. There are times when patients long for someone to listen to what they are carrying and what is troubling them. Retired schoolteacher Jim Mulcahy was carrying, to be sure, more than most. Besides a diagnosis of lymphoma, Jim's wife and three of his four children had been diagnosed with Huntington's disease. (His remarkable story can be found on the Canadian Virtual Hospice [virtualhospice.ca], *A Story About Care*.) Late one night while in hospital, Jim found himself unable to sleep, worrying about his cancer and what would become of his family. As scary thoughts and despair were doing their best to keep him awake, he tells the story of a nurse who came into his room during her ward rounds.

> An old nurse at the end of her career . . . "old nurse," she would probably swat me if she heard me say that, but she was let's say "mature," in the latter part of her career. As a matter of fact, she had 1 year to go in a career that stretched back over 35 years. She came in one night, and the evenings were long and hard, and she sat down in the one little chair that was beside my bed and took off her shoes and stretched out her feet. I can see her, and she sort of sighed and said, "I'm just going to talk with you for a while if you don't mind." It was the hollow of the night. A scary time for me and she talked; and she talked about her kids, and she let me talk about my kids, what I did as a profession, and asked me about those things, and it was wonderful, because she was addressing me as a complex individual who had a life, who had kids, who had a wife who worried about him. Not just my medical history but my personal history, and I just loved her for that. I just loved her for that.

Dr. Corneleus Woelk is a family physician and palliative care doctor with over 30 years of experience working in rural Manitoba. He describes some specific ways, depending on the clinical situation, of conveying the message "I am here to listen to you." When he does a home visit, for example, he says, "You take your shoes off at the door, because you're being respectful, and you take your time. And you listen. And you're willing to listen, even when they go down paths that you think, well, we don't really need to talk about that; you still talk about that. You follow their lead and ride their wave for a while." He describes a different approach for patients being seen in clinic or in hospital, particularly when he anticipates challenging communication issues.

> My nurses know that when I walk with them into an exam room and I pull out and sit down on the footstool, that I'm doing that for a reason. It's very hard for somebody to look down at their doctor and continue to be angry; and it's also a message that I'm willing to listen, and you can be up there, and I'm going to be down here now for a little while. Most of the time, it doesn't matter what level we sit at;

the doctor knows more medical details and can take control of the situation. But allowing the patient some control makes a difference. I did this a little while ago with a family that was unhappy, in general, and they were unhappy with some of the steps along the way. The family physician had missed this, and then the oncologist had told them that, and now the surgeon was telling them something else, and "why can't you guys get things together." I knew ahead of time that that this was going to be a difficult encounter, and I had to somehow give the patient and the family a little more control. He had a pancreatic cancer that was initially probably missed. These cancers can be difficult to diagnose early, and then, by the time they get caught, we're kind of too late. In this case, rightly or wrongly, they blamed the system and various people within the system for the late diagnosis. So, I walked into the room with the nurse, and I immediately knew that this was going to be difficult. You know how you can just feel it sometimes? You walk into a room and say to yourself "this isn't going to go well." I'm not sure whether it's the air in the room, whether it's the way they look at you or something else. But I just reached my foot out, pulled the little footstool closer to me and sat down on it. And the nurse didn't bat an eye because she knew. Maybe I was sitting in a part of the air that was lighter. The whole room just felt a whole lot better. I don't know how I learnt to do that. Nobody taught me. Probably on one occasion there had just not been enough chairs in the room, I sat down on the footstool, and I realized, oh my goodness, the air is so much lighter down here.

Eye contact conveys a similar message. "I am here to see you." Patients need to be heard and seen. Lack of eye contact, on the other hand, can feel like the epitome of *failure to see or acknowledge* your patient and denial of personhood. Jill Taylor-Brown recalls a patient telling her, "that sometimes she felt like the nurse was attending to the machines more than she was attending to her. That so much attention went into checking that the IV was running right, but never looking her in the eye and making eye contact." Imagine an encounter with a medical receptionist or a triage nurse, perhaps someone entering a hospital room to deliver food or clean a room. It could be a physician or a nurse, really anyone working in healthcare. Averting someone's gaze sends the message, "who you are isn't really any of my concern." In a state of relative well-being, most of us can shake this off and treat it as little more than a minor, soon to be forgotten, annoyance. But people in need of healthcare are usually unwell or particularly vulnerable and, in the context of sickness or fear, can be exquisitely sensitive.

Even tiny nuances can cause someone to suddenly feel that they don't matter, that they have figuratively disappeared. An elderly hospitalized woman, regal in appearance as I recall, told me how she took exception to the fact that a junior staff member *had the gall* to call her by her first name. As it happened, she had been a professional in her own right, and the assumption that someone would address her so casually made her feel devalued and unappreciated. Not being afforded the courtesy of being addressed more formally as "doctor" made her feel that part of her was being overlooked and somehow repudiated. Another story of *failure to see* comes from a wonderful geriatrician, Dr. Colin Powell. Dr. Powell was Professor and Head of the Division of Geriatric Medicine, Department of Medicine, Dalhousie University and Director of the Centre for Health Care of the Elderly at Queen Elizabeth II Health Sciences Centre in Halifax Nova Scotia. He described a consultation he had been asked to provide on an elderly gentleman living in a personal care home for veterans. This resident had some moderate cognitive impairment associated with dementia and recent behavioral dyscontrol. Upon reviewing the chart Dr. Powell discovered that, hidden within the psychosocial history, this gentleman had been a highly decorated Canadian soldier. As part of his therapeutic intervention, he informed the staff of this discovery and advised them that, henceforth, the patient should be referred to by his formal military titles, Lieutenant Commander. In very short order, the behavioral problems began to settle down.

Behavior and Elderspeak

A common mode of *failure to see the patient* in seniors is so-called *elderspeak*. Elderspeak is a way of behaving and a fashion of speaking with older persons that assumes their lack of competence. Using collective plural pronouns—for example, "Are we ready for our bath?"—implies the person's inability to make choices or decisions independently. Similarly, tag questions, such as "You want to get up now, don't you?" are designed to bend people to a particular outcome or singular choice. Then there are infantilizing forms of address, which use inappropriately intimate terms such as "sweetie," "honey," "good girl," or "dear." This approach insists upon seeing the elderly through a generic and saccharine lens. This pseudo-affectionate way of referring to seniors essentially says, "Your name is not important to me. You are all the same." If everyone deserves to be called "sweetie" or "dear," one might assume that it is plausible that no one merits that designation, that, in effect, those words come from a place that is indifferent and disingenuous.

Studies on elderspeak provide ample testimony of how people respond when they are treated with such *failure to see* indifference. One study found a causal relationship between elderspeak and resistiveness to care in older adults with dementia. This study reported that older adults with dementia most frequently reacted to elderspeak with negative vocalizations such as screaming, yelling, or crying. Conversely, reducing elderspeak saw improvements in quality of care to these residents.[9] Other researchers have drawn an association between elderspeak and negative self-perceptions, which they report have been linked with more negative images of aging and worse functional health over time, including lower rates of survival. In a long-term survey of 660 people older than 50, researchers found that those who had positive perceptions of aging lived an average of 7.5 years longer, a bigger increase than that associated with exercising or not smoking.[10] These findings held up even when the researchers controlled for differences in the participants' health conditions.

Behavior, Embarrassment, and Shame

Being human means being vulnerable. Recall the Latin derivative of vulnerability means "to wound" and that *everyone* is susceptible to being wounded by way of illness or injury. Besides being induced by sick or injured bodies, vulnerability can be heightened or provoked by how healthcare providers behave toward patients. Obtaining healthcare requires yielding power and control. Things people normally keep private and hidden from almost everyone must now be revealed, examined, and probed. The circumstances of this kind of scrutiny happen because of apprehension about the integrity or functioning of the body. Just as the body is declaring its wayward agenda and asserting control, patients must expose themselves to the critical gaze of a healthcare provider whose role is to take charge and determine what is going on and what options there are for what can or should be done about it.

Relinquishing control, yielding power, deferring to the authority of others, all add up to a diminished sense of personal autonomy. Particularly in Western culture, autonomy is often conflated with personhood, core identity, and self-worth. Hence an assault on autonomy is often experienced as an assault on the essence of life itself. Despite a profound desire to be in control, wayward bodies can transport us into the realm of human experience well beyond the purview of unshattered autonomy. Imagine a young toddler acting out in a crowded bus. All eyes turn toward this unpleasant scene as the parents feel mounting embarrassment, anger, and helplessness in addition to feeling judged and, for the time, being stuck. Despite the best of parenting, toddlers sometimes misbehave. So, too, is the case with bodies. Despite the best of care and through no fault of our own, bodies sometimes misbehave. When they do, bodies draw unwanted attention and cause us to feel fallible, responsible, and embarrassed. Unlike the scenario of the wayward children, there is no getting off at the next stop. There is simply no way of leaving our body behind or disassociating ourselves from its current acting out in ways that are beyond our control. Losing bowel or bladder control, losing the ability to think clearly, losing functional capacity or mobility, any of these scenarios can be mortifying. To "mortify" means to cause abject embarrassment and comes from the Latin, *mortificare*, which means *to cause death*. Little wonder that anticipating loss of autonomy is often perceived as a fate worse than death.

Shame can be a painful counterpoint to embarrassment. Embarrassment describes a feeling of discomfort in having been seen to violate a social rule or norm. It is situational and fluctuates, depending on its cause and who is there to take notice. Embarrassment requires a witness. Shame on the other hand describes a feeling of discomfort that is borne internally, wherein you are your own witness and punitive judge. Embarrassment sounds like "You make me feel bad. You make me feel weak." Whereas shame sounds like, "I am bad. I am weak." Many years ago, I looked after a young man with metastatic testicular cancer. The referral came because the medical oncologist was concerned about how this patient was responding to his illness. Despite a seemly stable relationship with his common-law girlfriend, he precipitously decided to move out, not wanting her to witness his *less than manly* descent into cancer treatment, which he feared might render him less than whole. "If I can't be the guy who carries the groceries into our apartment, she's better off without me." He felt embarrassed to be seen by friends and family, concerned that they would see him as less than his previous self. And he felt shame, convinced that he *was weak*, that he *was fragile*, that he *was* no longer worthy of his girlfriend's affections and no longer the person he had once been.

Being a Witness

Working in healthcare means bearing witness to our patients' experiences, experiences that are often marked by vulnerability, uncertainty, and fear. Being a skilled and reliable witness means considering myriad evidence before arriving at definitive clinical conclusions. Being a skillful witness requires being ever mindful of assumptions or biases that can influence how we perceive patients, whether based on attitudes toward aging, culture, religion, social status, sexual orientation, gender, weight/size, class, or disability. For patients, our failure to do so can feel like a disavowal of who they are and what they are going through and risks them feeling misunderstood or feeling that aspects of their experience have not been adequately seen, appreciated, or acknowledged.

As witnesses we are in a position to do much good, but we also have the power to cause great harm. The task of a skillful witness is to see as much as possible and to affirm truth. Conversely, failure to see truth or seeing a distortion of truth or only a partial truth—bearing false witness—can hurt patients. Healthcare professionals pride themselves on being able to sift through evidence, including patients' histories, symptoms, examinations, and test results, and reach their verdict, expressed in terms of diagnostic pronouncements and treatment decisions. We spend our professional lives honing the ability to see and evaluate patients based on various medical parameters and objective criteria. "Patient" is a generic label, based not on who the person is, but the ailment they are afflicted with. Little wonder that patients sometimes loathe these clinical, impersonal designations, reducing them to signs, symptoms, and diagnoses, threatening to usurp their identity, their perception of themselves, and how they imagine others see and appreciate the totality of who they are as human beings.

The most abject distortion of being a witness, failure to see the humanity in others, underscores most human rights violations, violations that disavow the basic tenet of the Universal Declaration of Human Rights. "All human beings are born free and equal in dignity and rights. They are endowed with reason and conscience and should act toward one another in a spirit of brotherhood." The word "dignity" comes from the Latin *dignitatem* or *dignitas* meaning *worthiness*, or *dignus* meaning *worth*. Hence dignity is the inherent and inalienable worth of all human beings irrespective of age, social status, race, ethnicity, religion, gender, sexual orientation, or physical or mental state. Within the clinical arena, violations of dignity are most often associated with a perception of *not being seen*.[3] Understandable, given that dignity itself refers to being deserved of honor, respect, or esteem. *Failure to see* can feel like a repudiation of personhood, a sense of lacking in worth, and a fracturing of sense of dignity. Dr. Bruce Martin says that "some of the most skilled people I've encountered in my career are those who were certain about things like tumors, abnormal lab tests, but took every bit as much interest in the patient and his or her life journey."

Within healthcare, a witness not only takes in patient experience, but is a critical part of that experience. Recall that sensing embarrassment requires a witness. In other words, a witness is no mere passive observer, but also a key player within this dynamic; a player whose disposition shapes the patient's subjective response to their healthcare circumstance. So, for instance, being a skillful witness in healthcare means mitigating actions, reactions, or behaviors that might cause embarrassment or cause the patient to feel diminished. This does not mean pretending that patients are not weakened or fragile or vulnerable, but behaving in a fashion that shows we understand those things to be a feature of their condition and not a reflection of their worth.

Respecting boundaries and safeguarding privacy are critical elements of being a skillful witness. While examining naked bodies and probing orifices may be routine within the realm of clinical medicine, there is nothing routine about this when your body and orifices are the subject of scrutiny. To be naked means not only to lack clothing, but also to lack protection, which is the essence of vulnerability. The word "palliative" comes from the Latin *palliare*, which means *to cover with a cloak* or *to conceal*. As witnesses we prevent harm by asking permission to perform examinations, by only exposing bodies to the degree required, and by providing *a cloak*, hence covering fragile bodies and soothing frayed nerves.

I recall one morning, several decades ago, being a medical student taking part in morning ward rounds as part of my rotation on internal medicine. As memory serves me, there were about six trainees in all that day, residents and medical students, under the supervision of an attending internist. These rounds were being run pretty efficiently, with each of us being asked to present our patients to the attending as we made our way from room to room in this particular hospital ward. We eventually found ourselves in the room of an older man, who as I recall had myriad health problems, including some moderate degree of cognitive impairment. Given that this gentleman was quite placid, our attending decided that this would be the perfect occasion for each of us to practice doing a rectal examination. I do not recall the patient being asked his permission to take part in this educational escapade, nor do I recall any protest from him as each student lined up to take their turn. As I recall, I was the last person in the room. Whether I have forgotten or choose to forget if I performed the examination is moot. What I do remember, all these years later, are the tears I noticed rolling down his cheek as I took leave of him and exited his room.

C Stands for Compassion

Compassion refers to the awareness of the suffering of another, accompanied by the wish to respond to it. The Latin root for the word compassion is *pati*, which means *to suffer*, and the prefix *com*, meaning *with*. Compassion, originating from *compati*, literally means *to suffer with*. Compassion implicates both how we feel and how we respond toward patients. While there is little doubt that most people working in healthcare would purport to value compassion and all its associated virtues, in truth, very little time, education, and resources are invested in prioritizing and implementing compassionate outlooks and practices. Compassion is what separates *healthcare* from *healthcaring*. Healthcare systems are organized around the delivery of evidence-based medicine and are focused on providing skills and services that are largely technical and knowledge-based. Healthcaring, that is healthcare imbued with compassion, implicates not only what we do with or for patients, but also ways of being with and acting toward patients.

Take the case of Mrs. J., a 47-year-old woman, mother of three teenagers, with metastatic breast cancer. The treatments and approaches she was offered were formulaic, determined and justified based on the outcomes of national and international randomized, peer-reviewed, clinical trials. Based on those studies, her oncologist arranged a course of radiation therapy, a perfectly justifiable approach given her current symptomatology and the extent to which her disease had spread. She arrived at her appointment, having been told it was for simulation. *Simulation* is a procedure done prior to starting a patient on radiation therapy, which carefully determines the fields that are to be radiated. Mrs. J. had been told that she would have to lie very still in a special immobilization device on the treatment table. She also understood that pictures would be taken of the area that needed to be treated and that those pictures would be sent to a radiation planning computer to determine the exact treatment fields, which are the areas of the breast to be radiated. However, what she had not been told was that once the treatment fields were set, the radiation oncologist would mark out the corners of the field with a felt pen. Not understanding why this was being done, and having had no forewarning, Mrs. J. said she felt "like a slab of meat, like a piece of paper." Indeed, she was so distraught because of this experience, she considered withdrawing from treatment altogether. Although she ultimately decided in favor of continuing, she remained distrustful and frightened throughout the remainder of her radiation.

To be clear, Mrs. J.'s healthcare, in terms of the appropriateness of what treatment she was offered and the technical competence with which it was delivered, were beyond reproach. But there was an element of *healthcaring* that sadly fell short, leaving her feeling dehumanized and objectified. Surely there was no malicious intent whatsoever on the part of her healthcare providers, who, without being told how she felt, would have assumed that they had carried out their task impeccably. Anticipating her healthcare needs and experience through a lens of compassion requires trying to think about Mrs. J. as a person and what this illness and this treatment might mean to her; how the process of preparing for radiation, being naked, having to position her body to facilitate the accurate passage of radiation, being drawn on, might make her—or any patient, for that matter—feel.

Healthcaring, seeing patients through a lens of compassion, requires that we ask, "How might this make someone feel?" Asking this question shifts the frame of reference, changing the way clinicians perceive and respond to patients. It also shifts the care tenor—those ineffable emotional and empathic qualities of a clinical encounter shaped by the healthcare provider. Healthcaring insists that attending to the needs of the patient goes hand in hand with sensitivity to the patient's feelings. To be sure, healthcaring will not eliminate all the toils of patienthood (case in point, radiation fields still need to be marked). But applying the lens of healthcaring— "How might this make someone feel?"—changes the tone of care, eliciting clear explanations, perhaps a gentle touch, a kind word, or an understanding look. Healthcaring is ever mindful that *patients are people with feelings that matter.* Those feelings almost always include a heightened sense of vulnerability, dependency, and loss of control, which can be internally driven by the underlying condition but also externally imposed (depending on the nature and tone of the health care encounter), resulting in threatened self-efficacy and fractured personhood. Dr. Robert Lotocki is a gynecological oncologist with more than three decades of clinical experience at CancerCare Manitoba. He points out that "whatever happens to the cancer, we must realize that patients are human beings. They are not a CancerCare number. They have got a name and they have a history and a personality, and, unfortunately, they also have cancer."

There are times when compassion means being physically present in the face of suffering. Dr. Pam Orr is Professor of Internal Medicine, Medical Microbiology and Community Health Sciences at the University of Manitoba. She has been practicing medicine for nearly 45 years. She recalled, "a 28-year-old woman from South Africa who was dying of AIDS in the hospital. These were bad times for HIV, when there was no treatment. She had a 10-year-old son but no other family support, no friends, no colleagues, and she was on the general medical ward. I came in and the nurse told me she was dying. I sat with her and basically held her hand, because I felt that was the care she required or I imagined she required. She was not very responsive, but I sat with her, holding her hand for nearly 2 hours. Nearly 25 years later, I still remember that it was a Sunday, very busy, and people running around. The nurse peeked around the corner and she looked at me and I looked at her, and she seemed a little embarrassed as if she had intruded on something private, and I felt a little embarrassed because I knew this wasn't very common. Years later I ran into that nurse, who told me while she thought it was unusual, that it was a good thing to do."

Seeing Patients Through a Compassionate Lens

Some healthcare providers are intuitively compassionate. They seem to have an innate ability to recognize their patients' suffering and to be moved by it; that is, they are moved to feel and respond. For these people, compassion seems reflexive and automatic. Dr. Harlos is one such person, although he would qualify this by pointing out that not every situation elicits the same reaction. Like most people, the more a clinical encounter approximates a reality we can recognize, personalize, or conjure up in our mind's eye, the more easily our capacity for compassion is realized. For instance, Dr. Harlos described a house call he made to see a dying 18-year-old. "I'd never met him before nor met the family. So, I drive into his little neighborhood and see all these kids playing on the side of the street." Dr. Harlos happens to be the father of three young grown children, and he finds himself thinking, "Five years ago, that was him—this patient I'm about to see." He then turns up the driveway to the house: "I notice a basketball hoop on the garage and know that that was his." By now the feelings and the associations are inescapable. "I was met at the door by the parents. You just cannot imagine sadder looking people and once in the house, there are basketball shoes sitting at the doorway, which are his, but will never be worn again. And then there are the pictures on the wall of graduation, which makes it very hard to find your balance."

The balance Dr. Harlos is referring to is a dynamic equilibrium that all clinicians must negotiate—the emotional balancing act that teeters between feeling overwhelmed by the emotional intensity of a given clinical encounter and the defensive inclination to emotionally disconnect. "It always makes me think of a surfer on a wave. If you get too close, you crash. But if you get too far back behind the wave, you've lost it. Walking in that home, the wave just got a little rougher, a little bit bigger. So, you are having to work harder to strike the right balance."

Jill Taylor-Brown recalled a patient describing being very sick with an infection and telling her about a nurse, "who at some point started to cry and say to the patient, 'I'm sorry that I can't take better care of you. I've been working 14 hours straight because my colleagues haven't come in.'" Clearly either extreme, that is, emotional disengagement or feeling emotionally overwhelmed, is problematic and can undermine good patient care. Getting too close, like inching toward a fire, can burn you. The patient's tragedy and the family's angst become internalized. You see yourself and the people you love in their circumstances, rendering you emotionally spent and therapeutically ineffective. On the other hand, if you keep yourself too far distant, you may be able to carry out the technical and practical elements of healthcare but not be able to make an authentic and comforting therapeutic connection. Says Dr. Harlos, "You have to be close enough to feel at least a little bit of heat."

There are other instances when compassion feels less intuitive and needs some encouragement. Linda works in a radiation oncology clinic. These clinics can be tough, in that patients are almost always very sick and being radiated for painful bony metastasis or receiving radiation for leukemia, lymphomas, or germ cell tumors. Radiation is commonly used to treat solid tumors, such as head and neck cancer, breast cancer, non–small cell lung cancer, cervical cancer, anal cancer, and prostate cancer. Within any given cancer center, patients must vie for a limited number of radiation machines that are scheduled throughout the course of a day. Imagine the pressure on the radiation oncology clerks who must respond to patients' requests for when their treatment will be slotted, particularly given that the number of machines and the hours they operate are entirely beyond their control.

Linda is an experienced radiation oncology clerk, experienced enough to know the challenges of trying to accommodate all varieties of patients' requests. She admitted that there were days when these inquires felt like demands and expressed how frustrating it could be to find herself on the receiving end of dissatisfaction, trying to resolve many problems well beyond her control. One day during a busy clinic she recounted being approached by an elderly gentleman with a scheduling request. Although the words were barely out of his mouth, she could feel her irritation and annoyance mounting. His demeanor, however, seemed kind, and he did not strike her as entitled, brash, or demanding. Those initial impressions caused her to take a moment, swallow her irritation, and ask him why he needed the time slot he had requested for his radiation treatment. He responded by telling Linda that his wife had Alzheimer's disease, and, although they still managed to live together in their small apartment, his wife needed almost constant supervision. For the past year home care was spelling him off for a few hours each morning. Hence, so long as he could get his treatments during that interval, he and his wife were still able to manage.

Linda described her response to this disclosure as transformative. His request no longer felt like a demand, but rather a perfectly reasonable arrangement that would accommodate his needs and his wife's needs as well. While she admitted to initially assuming his reasons for wanting to be slotted into morning appointments might be frivolous and arbitrary, his explanation struck her as well-grounded, selfless, even noble, given that the timing for his treatment was in the service of him looking after his ailing life partner. This quality of transformation speaks directly to how differently things can look through the lens of compassion. By virtue of his response, her perception of this man had changed, as did her feelings toward him. Recall that compassion is a two-sided coin, with one side implicating how we understand our patients suffering and the flip side being what we do with those feelings by way of responding to our patients. Knowing this man was attempting to fulfill his role as a faithful husband and care provider, values that struck a chord with Linda, moved her to enthusiastically do everything within her ability to accommodate his request.

Compassion can sometimes feel hard, particularly when there are barriers that thwart our attempts to mitigate suffering. Jill Taylor-Brown described one occasion in which her efforts drove her to tears. "I remember crying in my office. I was just so frustrated. I was trying to get childcare for a young mom who was having treatment and the person I was talking to in the social agency providing childcare was being rude and dismissive, and not helping me get for this client the care she needed for her child. I was so frustrated and felt so helpless. This poor mom is having chemotherapy. She can't look after her kids, and I can't get any help for her. I wasn't actually crying about this woman being on chemo because I have no control over that or that she has cancer and has to have chemo. But surely to God as a society we ought to be able to have things in place so we can care for her children while she is having treatment. The fact I couldn't make that happen and was talking to someone who was not helping me make that happen was just sending me over the top."

Sometimes compassion can be mindfully stoked. I recall, for instance, being on call one weekend for our Department of Psychiatry. Call could sometimes be harrowing, given the uncertainty of who might show up in emergency, what issues might come up on the wards, and what critical decisions might fall into your lap any given moment. This particular weekend, call had been busy. I had just walked into the psychiatry building after completing the consultations in ER. Two large security guards were forcibly moving a patient, a woman who was obviously floridly psychotic, up the entry flight of stairs enroute to the ward. Besides her shouting profanities, she had made her body as rigid as possible, forcing her guards to bodily carry her up each and every step.

Perhaps my own fatigue and preoccupation with the previous cases and decisions made earlier that day were still on my mind. As I watched this terrible ordeal unfold, I found myself feeling annoyed, impatient, and wishing I were anywhere else. But trying to get past that, and having little else to do but watch and follow from behind, I began wondering who this patient was and what her story might be. And while that would have to wait until I could read her chart or ask her directly, I began thinking about how it might feel to be so utterly out of control and emotionally unraveled. It then occurred to me that making her body rigid and cussing were the only forms of resistance available to her. While there was no question that she would soon end up on the locked psychiatric unit, the only part of this scenario that she could control was the ease with which that would be accomplished. And so she protested in the only way she new how, by not cooperating, by refusing to walk, and refusing to remain silence. As strange as it may seem, these thoughts found me feeling less annoyed and even admiring the strength it took to mount this sad albeit futile protest.

Compassion and Connecting the Pieces

Sinclair et al.[11] define compassion as *a virtuous response that seeks to address the suffering and needs of a person through relational understanding and action.*

What does this mean in day-to-day clinical practice, and how does one achieve it?

1. *Compassion begins by acknowledging the person who is suffering.* If we fail to see our patients as persons, it is easier to overlook their suffering and remain oblivious to things that cause, and ways they express, their suffering.
2. *Acknowledging patients as persons requires openness to their stories.* While patients have symptoms, persons have stories. While the former is generic and largely objective, the latter is completely individual and wholly subjective and experiential. Openness to stories means being willing to see and know what makes each person feel unique.
3. *Broaching personhood means accepting vulnerability.* By coming to know or appreciate the patient as a person, we become aware of the human drama in which the illness takes place. This context includes relationships, history, culture, beliefs, principles, vocation, interests, and whatever else might define a persons' essence. Being drawn into their stories (i.e., *relational understanding*) and feeling a resonance with their stories, creates a mutual sense of vulnerablity and shared humanity.
4. *Accepting personal vulnerability sets the stage for compassionate caring.* Hearing patients' stories that include critical elements of who they are allows healthcare providers to relate in ways that are personal and affecting.

5. To feel compassion, *to suffer with*, means to understand that, like your patients, you, too, are vulnerable and mortal, and those fundamental dimensions of human experience unfold within a life story that, like your patient's, is unique and finite.
6. Compassion requires a virtuous response; that is, action intended to mitigate the patient's suffering.

Dr. Gingerich recalled a case wherein knowing the patient's story and being moved toward a virtuous response demonstrated the epitome of compassionate care.

A few years ago, I was asked to see a young man in his 20s with metastatic colorectal cancer. The question was whether any more chemotherapy would be helpful to him. Unfortunately, there wasn't any other chemotherapy available for him, but we started talking about his story, which was an extremely sad situation. He was from the Philippines and his wife and child had moved from the Philippines to Canada before him, and he was back at home making money and paying to support them and trying to make enough money for him to come join them. It took a number of months until he finally got enough money to come. As soon as he landed in Winnipeg, his wife met him at the airport and said that she didn't want to see him anymore, that she'd met someone else and didn't want anything to do with him and didn't want him to see his daughter. So he was all by himself in Winnipeg and soon after his arrival, he began having cancer symptoms and was diagnosed with metastatic disease. He had nowhere to stay, didn't know anyone, and had this new diagnosis of advanced cancer. He eventually found some fellow Filipinos that were able to care for him and take him under their wings and gave him food and a place to live while he was undergoing treatment. Eventually the chemotherapy stopped working, he became more symptomatic, which is why I was asked to see him in the hospital.

While there wasn't anything more to do about curing his cancer, we worked on his symptoms. It was clear that he was dying and didn't have much time left and no family or anybody around to be with him for the end. He mentioned to me that his most important goal was to have his mom come and see him before he died, and his mom lived in the Philippines. The way he worded it, he was crying when he said this, was, "Can you promise me that you'll help me get my mom here before I die." I remember thinking that I didn't know how I was going to respond to that because that's a bit out of my control. I really can't promise something like that, so I said I would try and do everything I could to help with the process. It was a pretty emotional interaction. A lot of what happened wouldn't have come out of it had I just focused on the medical part of it. I wrote letters to the embassy and the Manitoba government because they needed a special visa to get the mom here. Then there was a financial component to it, and the team that was taking care of him in the hospital and his friends in the Winnipeg community got together to raise money for his mother to come to Canada. Eventually, they were able to raise enough money and get all the approvals in place for her to come.

It took a couple of weeks, but she flew in and made it. I remember walking into the room after she had arrived, she was in the room with him, and he was eating a home-cooked meal that she had prepared for him that was his favorite meal, and he had this huge smile on his face. It was actually quite powerful, and although his suffering and symptoms were still there, it seemed to me they had come down a notch. He died soon after. It was all pretty powerful.

D Stands for Dialogue

Medicine is full of conversations, with much of the dialogue dominated by complex technical issues, specialty nomenclature, and jargon and language designed to describe objective realities of illness and illness experience. "D for Dialogue", however, refers to a different kind of discourse, one that acknowledges, affirms, or otherwise broaches some aspect of personhood. These conversations need not be lengthy or time-consuming and can be seamlessly interwoven into whatever the illness or disease-specific clinical agenda happens to be. Take the example of Dr. James Johnston. Dr. Johnston is a very fine and caring medical oncologist specializing in hematological malignancies at CancerCare Manitoba. His practice is busy, and his clinical pace is intense. I recall passing by his clinic one day as the door to the examination room he was entering was about to close. The last thing I heard before the door shut was, "so, how was that family vacation you went on?" It was a simple question, utterly disconnected from issues pertaining to the lymphoma, perhaps, that brought the patient to Dr. Johnston's attention. Given the number of people passing through his clinic, there is little doubt that the *vacation conversation* was brief, but, in those moments, it acknowledged that while lymphoma does not take a vacation, people do.

Taking Time to Hear the Person's Story

Clinicians are often reluctant to broach matters pertaining to personhood, fearing the amount of time it will take to do so. Dr. Martin indicates that making a connection need not be overly time-consuming. "I'm not talking about hours, but just a little bit of training and a few good, scripted questions so that they get the context, and they can build the confidence and trust and relationship with the patient. In training we don't allow the humanism to come out. I don't think we beat it out of them. I think we just don't elevate it to the point where it is seen to be terribly important. I had a mentor that talked to me about what you do in the first 15 seconds when you're in somebody's house. It's making sure you elevate discovering who this person is, just as we would the review of systems. So, if you see a patient who's a little bit blue and a little bit short of breath and you can hear their wheeze, you know what questions you're going to ask next. It's not much different than seeing a picture of a young lad standing in a military uniform with his hand on the propeller of an aircraft, leading you to saying, "so tell me about your life as a pilot."

Jill Taylor-Brown reflected on the importance of knowing each patient's story. "I've listened to hundreds and hundreds of stories. Yet each story is unique, and being side by side with them through these experiences has just become a part of me. When someone is in front of me and saying something, I'm hearing other people having spoken about these things. It is like they are somehow with me." In reflecting on dignity-conserving dialogue and notions of personhood, she recalled how patients sometimes spoke of *feeling invisible, like an inanimate object* that, while present, is not really seen. She described how patients often feel that more attention is being paid to their chart than to them, with clinicians not ever making eye contact or asking, "How are you doing?" These kinds of conversations don't necessarily have to be elaborate or extensive but, at a minimum, need to somehow make patients feel visible. "How are you holding up? This must be so difficult on you? Is that a photograph of your family? Can you introduce me to your visitors? Tell me what's been on your mind?"

I recall seeing an elderly gentleman over 35 years ago for psychiatric consultation because of some vague difficulties he was having with confusion. The clinical details of that encounter have long since faded into an amalgam of many similar such cases. I do, however, remember asking this gentleman about a photograph embossed on a coffee-cup on his bedside table, with a picture of a young man with an owl perched on his shoulder. He told me the story of how, nearly 70 years earlier, he had nursed this injured bird back to health and the photograph that was snapped as he was about to release it back into the wild. The memory of this story, and even a clear visual image of that photograph, affirms that conversations such as these can leave an indelible mark.

Some stories are more complicated than others, just as some lives are more complicated than others, and without knowing the patient's story, healthcare takes place in the absence of knowing the critical personal context. Tom Roche recalled a middle-aged woman with cancer, "whose whole life experience had been one of loss of various kinds. She had experienced abuse as a child. She had done therapy and had done very well, in the sense that she had been able to function in a job, had become a professional, had married, and had some children. But when she was diagnosed with cancer, a lot of the feeling that she had around the abuse came back. And it just wasn't the abuse, but also the neglect. She had been abused by a family member. It wasn't a parent, and she had a sense of being totally alone with that, not being able to go to her mother or her father or to anybody else to speak about this. Not being able to reach out for some kind of comfort in any way, and in some way having to carry this all of her life. In some way she also felt she was protecting her parents, who she felt were not terribly well, and she picked up on this, feeling she shouldn't disturb them, she shouldn't upset them, she should try to protect them when this horrible sequence of events happened to her. She felt unable to go to them for any kind of support and so was feeling very isolated and on her own. And what the cancer did was in some ways reawaken all the fear about being attacked, about being assaulted. And that's how she saw the cancer, even though it had been caught at an early stage and the prognosis seemed good. But there was this continual fear for a long time that 'it's going to come back. I'm going to be assaulted again by the cancer.'"

It seems inconceivable, in the absence of knowing something of this history and the nature of her outlook toward cancer, how one could provide person-centered dignity in care.

Conversations that acknowledge personhood, even in the smallest and seemingly inconsequential of ways, can change the care tenor of the clinical encounter. Similarly, failure to acknowledge personhood can undermine even the most seemingly flawless medical attention. As he was nearing his own death, Dr. Stewart Farber, a palliative care physician at the University of Washington, reflected on personhood and what he referred to as his *thread*.[12]

> With rare exception, the clinicians who treated me have good hearts, care deeply, but possess little or no knowledge of my thread. My thread is the narrative I use to make sense of my life. It is longitudinal, nonlinear, emotional, filled with contradictions, and integrates my life experiences into a coherent whole. It is within the values and meanings of my story that treatment decisions are made. What contributes to meaning and quality is not about living longer but living a life that is consistent with my thread. Without knowing my thread, it is impossible for a clinician to provide respectful care.

Denise Klassen is a clinical nurse at CancerCare Manitoba who has worked in oncology for nearly 20 years. In reflecting on the importance of knowing the patient's "thread" or story, she recalled a young woman with a localized pancreatic cancer.

> So obviously not someone who was curative and having to make a choice of either having more chemo or going a more conservative route and do palliative care. She decided to have more chemotherapy, which I think was a good decision. She was a single woman, who obviously had led a very, very rough life. When she came in the first day, I noticed when I did her blood pressure that she had hundreds of little slashes on her arms. She never wanted to take off her shirt for us to do any sort of abdominal exam, that was just off limits. One day she called me up and said she needed to read her story to me. "If I don't read it to you, I think I'll go back to becoming a binge drinker." I didn't realize she had quit drinking, so I said, okay, I'll give you half an hour. So she read me her story, but it meant the world to her. She said, over and over again, how much she appreciated that I had given her half an hour to simply hear her story. She walked away with a smile. She was on cloud nine, that she had been able to share parts of her life that she had kept hidden all of her life and how that somehow gave her the strength to keep going. She was a broken person and was not only dealing with her cancer, but also trying to figure out who she is, trying to put her life together for the time she had left, hopefully before her end of life. Subsequent to that appointment, she told me that she trusted me and allowed me to do an abdominal exam, but she wouldn't trust the doctor to do this, which made me wonder about a history of abuse.

When Dr. Harlos reflects on dialogue and personhood, he thinks about whole families. To illustrate this, he recalled the case of a 5-month-old girl born with a condition marked by rapidly progressive neuromuscular failure called *spinomuscular atrophy*.

> She presented to emergency with respiratory failure and was taken to the ICU. The parents decided that they were taking her home because, for them, personhood was that they were a family. This girl was born at home and the mom wanted her to die at home. The mom referred to the room as "the portal" afterwards, saying this is where her daughter came into this world, and where she will leave this world. Pediatric ICU had never had an experience with discharging someone home on noninvasive ventilatory support. She was admitted to ICU on a Wednesday, and we had her home by Friday on bi-level ventilation. We visited daily, sometimes more than once a day. The parents had a 2-year-old and a 5-year-old, siblings, two girls. They were all able to have little parties, dancing and eating pizza. They celebrated

every week as a milestone. She died at home in her mother's lap as she sang her daughter her favorite song. Afterward the mother was interviewed by a television show doing a piece on pediatric palliative care. She said that palliative care "couldn't save our daughter, but in the end they saved our family."

So what does it take to know a patient's *thread*, and how can clinicians enter into dialogue designed to explore and reveal elements of that thread? Sometimes just taking a few moments to acknowledge who the patient is and what is important to them makes all the difference. Dr. Lotocki finds that "for patients with overian cancer, paracentesis is a good time to sit down at their bedside, and, while you do the technical task of taking the fluid off, you are talking to the person. You might talk about the weather, or about their family interactions. So this gives you an opportunity to come back at the end of the day and see the patient when everyone else is gone, and talk to them personally."

Carolyn Jardine was a patient representative at CancerCare Manitoba. She recalls the case of an 80-year-old woman admitted to hospital, "with some kind of fracture to her spine in addition to a heart condition. It was extremely painful to move her because she had this fracture. We were struggling to help her. She was completely difficult to work with, upset and crying and feeling like we were giving her bad care. We called in a first-year resident and told him he had to do something for this lady. We were suggesting big-guns pain relief, like a shot of Fentanyl when we turned her. This resident sat down at the bedside and talked with her for not even 5 minutes. He brushed her hair, asked her about her kids and grandkids, and then explained why she was having such pain and got her to realize that if she moved in a certain way, that it wouldn't hurt as much. We ended up not even needing to give her much medication for the rest of the night. It really brought down her anxiety. She felt like this doctor was going to keep an eye on her and make sure that tomorrow morning things were taken care of. It really changed the whole way we took care of this patient." Being known instills a sense of trust and feeling cared for or, more to the point, feeling cared about. As this case illustrates, caring goes a long way toward alleviating physical as well as psychological distress.

The Patient Dignity Question and Acknowledging Personhood

Medicine is sometimes characterized as impersonal and routinized, with little attention paid to issues of personhood. This is often blamed on mounting time pressures and emphasis on delivering evidence-based quality health-care. However, a lack of caring can undermine trust and jeopardize the quality of the patient–healthcare provider relationship. This can impede pa-tient disclosures and lead to misdiagnoses, lack of clarity around the goals of care, and compromised patient safety. In such instances, patients and families are more likely to feel that their real concerns have not been heard, acknowl-edged, or addressed, increasing the likelihood of complaints or even litiga-tion. Disengagement from the caring facets of medicine is also associated with healthcare provider burnout and clinical ineffectiveness.

Acknowledgment of personhood should be foundational within the culture of medicine. And yet broaching this aspect of patient experience is often done with trepidation, with concerns that it may be too time-consuming or too emotionally evocative for patients and healthcare providers alike. However, failure to acknowledge personhood, seeing people in terms of their ailment rather than who they are, is often at the root of patient and family dissatisfac-tion and why medicine is sometimes perceived as uncaring or emotionally abrasive.

In order to facilitate conversations that elicit personhood, our research group developed the Patient Dignity Question (PDQ), which asks patients or those speaking on their behalf, *What do I need to know about you/your family member as a person to give you/them the best care possible?*[13] Because the PDQ prompts information regarding personhood, it enhances dignity by way of changing healthcare provider perception regarding who their patients are as persons. The conversations elicited are meant to be no more than 10–15 minutes. They often begin with a statement to the effect, "although I know a lot about who you are as a patient, I know much less about who you are as a person." This is then followed by posing the PDQ: "What should I (your healthcare provider) know about you (your family member) as a person to give you (them) the best care possible?" Respondents are given an opportu-nity to reflect on their answer or ask for clarification, with various prompts to further elicit a conversation focused on personhood: "What would you want any staff member walking into this room to know about you/them as a person? Do you have special qualities you would want them to see? Are there key roles or relationships you would want them to know about? Are there specific concerns, or important beliefs, you would want them to be aware of?"

Once these responses were completed, they were summarized by the re-search nurse into one to three paragraphs. These summaries were then read back to the participants, confirming that they were accurate, determining if any additions or deletions were required, and, if they agreed, having it placed on their medical chart. Afterall, if dignity is dependent on the perceptions of how one is perceived and appreciated, we anticipated that the PDQ would provide a lens through which patients would want to be seen.

The following are examples of PDQ responses elicited from patients receiving inpatient palliative care:[13]

Patient A: A 72-year-old married woman with end-stage metastatic breast cancer. A. jokes that there are three important things in her life, in this order: hair, family, and nails. This is A.'s way of saying that she is very particular, and always has been, about her personal appearance. She is a very proper person who does not want to be seen in public without perfect hair, make-up, and being well-dressed. Lipstick and a little rouge continue to be a must for her. But the most important thing is her hair. She likes it to be done and that her hairdo remains intact.

Personal cleanliness is also extremely important to A. and part of her morning and evening routine. She would appreciate being able to maintain this routine while in hospital, and, when she needs help, her preference would be to have a woman help her. A. can be very anxious. It is helpful if care providers explain what they are going to do before they do it. This would help her remain calm and not become short of breath. If she is experiencing pain, it is hard for her to be patient about waiting for medication.

Patient B: A 74-year-old divorced woman with end-stage lung cancer. B. feels her family has let her down. It has taken a long time, but she realizes that sometimes you cannot change people. She doesn't want her family anywhere around her. They are not wanted. She stresses the importance of confidentiality. "I do not want them to know anything about me."

Patient C: A 55-year-old divorced businesswoman with uterine cancer. C. describes herself as a mature, active, career-oriented corporate executive who gets the job done. An accomplished businesswoman, C. is accustomed to listening carefully to her clients and then creating and delivering solutions to their needs. She applies her own professionalism and business experience to the expectations she has of the healthcare system and her healthcare providers. She has taken an active learning role in the treatment of her illness and, therefore, expects a collaborative team approach from her caregivers, something she hears in words but does not always see in practice. Rather than being seen as a sick person needing help, C. would rather be viewed as a businesswoman fighting cancer with a goal of conquering it, whether that be conquering it on a physical level or on an emotional and psychological level. She wants to be given *an ear* for airing her concerns. She appreciated being cared for with dignity and respect.

Patient D: A 76-year-old separated woman with end-stage stomach cancer: On a practical note, D. says that her muscles and skin are very tender lately so she likes her caregivers to be very gentle when lifting or repositioning her. She also suggests patting rather than rubbing her skin when she is being bathed. D.'s appetite has been poor lately. She normally loves to eat. It bothers her when people coax her to eat. It's not that she doesn't want to eat, she just cannot. D. cautions her caregivers not to be offended if she says something inappropriate or hurtful. That's not really her, but her condition. D. likes that staff explain to her what they're going to do that day, or that they are going to try this or that. D. treasures coming to this hospital. Her mother was cared for and died here many years ago. D. says, "I feel like she's looking after me."

Patient E: A 64-year-old married woman with pancreatic cancer: E. acknowledges that her tough exterior hides a really soft interior. She says, "I am covering up so they cannot really see me." She says the way she talks is not meant to be disrespectful to anyone. Sometimes she's trying to hide the fact that she doesn't remember things and doesn't want to appear stupid. She says she used to have a memory like an elephant but not now. She calls everybody "sweetheart," "pumpkin," or "honeybunch" because she has a hard time remembering people's names. E. says she is scared. She lets everyone believe that she can handle it, that she's a trooper. She pretends everything is fine but it's not. It brings her to tears when she thinks about dying. She doesn't want to die. E. says she wants people to know she has these feelings, that although she tries to hide it, there is a storm brewing inside. She feels that if people know that's how she really feels then she will not have to put up a front anymore. She also wants to be told the truth right away.

Patient F: A 67-year-old married woman with metastatic lung cancer: A very important part of F.'s life is her Christian faith. She was raised in the Anglican Church. Her faith helps her face her terminal illness with honesty and peace. She believes that all the work God wanted her to do here on earth will be finished and that she will go in comfort knowing that she has done everything she wanted to do. Hearing the truth from the doctors is very important to F. so that she can face the problem head on. She does not want to be patronized.

Patient G: A 60-year-old divorced woman with lymphoma. G. finds it hard to trust but usually still does until something happens to change that trust. She says she wants to be independent and do as much as possible by herself. To that end, she would prefer that the people caring for her ask, "What can you do?" or "How do you usually do this?" as opposed to "we're going to do this." G. describes herself as a well-organized person, and this keeps things from getting overwhelming. It's important not to move things without asking her. G. needs to pace herself or she runs out of breath or gets pain. To help her pace herself and keep organized, it's important that healthcare providers ask her before they do something to or for her or assume they know what she would like done and how.

Family A: A is a 48-year-old daughter, responding to the PDQ for her 87-year-old father, H., who has myeloma. There are several characteristics that A. thinks are important for healthcare providers to know about her dad. He is a veteran of World War II and someone she describes as "truly a gentle giant." He's a person who puts the needs and wishes of others before his own. He can be easily persuaded and may go along with a person's suggestion although that may not be his preference. When someone asks him how he is, his tendency will be to respond with "I'm fine." If he is in pain, he may be reluctant to say so. He will not be forthcoming with problems unless you dig a little bit further. He just keeps it in and trudges along. A. observes that her dad also has some difficulty remembering. She is concerned that healthcare providers may be getting incorrect information. His answers may seem appropriate but after the healthcare provider leaves the room, he will acknowledge that he didn't really understand what was said.

Family B: B is the 40-year-old daughter of I., a 79-year-old widow with end-stage lung cancer. I. is a very modest person and is acutely uncomfortable with males giving her any intimate care. She is sensitive, and the discomfort she expressed regarding male caregivers was distressing and embarrassing for her as she felt misunderstood. Decreasing independence has been a real struggle for I. She can sometimes become a little "snippy" because she wants to do as much for herself as she can. She appreciates eye contact, partly because she is hard of hearing and the direct eye contact gives her visual cues. In the past few weeks, she has had an increased sensitivity to noise and cannot tolerate more than a couple of visitors at a time. As well, she is no longer able to watch TV or listen to music as she finds them too much stimulation. She has always appreciated things to be in order and tidy but now more than ever. I. loves touch like back and feet rubs, her face being washed, or hair being brushed. All these things calm her.

Family C: C. is the 65-year-old niece of her 100-year-old aunt, J. C. describes her aunt J. as a refined lady who is very particular and someone who likes things to be neat, tidy, and in order. J., who will be 101 in December, lived in her own beautiful apartment until just last week. She was very healthy until about 3 years ago. J. was born in Canada and left for the United States in 1928. For many years, J. worked in a beautiful boutique where they sold exclusive fashion to people like the Fords and the Dodges. J. is blind in her left eye. Her hearing is good. She has always had a lot of pain from osteoar-thritis so appreciates slow and gentle turning and moving. J. likes having her hair nicely combed, her face washed, and her teeth brushed.

These examples illustrate just how rich and telling responses to inquiries about personhood can be. Each one demonstrates facets of personhood that speak to the essence of who these patients are as people. The range of responses is vast and diverse, covering everything from the need to be touched gently or moved carefully in order to avoid pain and discomfort, not wanting to appear confused and vulnerable, having one's previous status or role in life acknowl-edged, to harboring fears of death itself. Attempting to provide holistic dignity in care in the absence of knowing this kind of information is akin to trying to navigate a complex maze when it is pitch black. As Dr. Gingerich affirms, "you need to realize that they are more than just a patient, they're a person and they have wants, needs, desires, and there's a whole part of them that you might not focus on if you are just looking at the medical part."

Over the course of our study, 126 PDQs were completed, 66 by patients and 60 by family members. The average age of patients was 74 years, with the ma-jority having some form of end-stage cancer and the remainder various non-malignant terminal conditions. Most of the family participants were women (74%) and included patients' spouses/partners, adult children, or siblings who generally knew the patient for a very long time (i.e., just under 50 years). Of the 126 PDQs, 98% of participants agreed or strongly agreed that the summa-ries were accurate, 96% gave permission to have them placed on the medical chart, 75% wanted a copy, 85% felt the information was important for HCPs to know, 64% felt it could affect care, and 92% indicated they would recommend it for others in their circumstances.

The PDQ study also evaluated how healthcare providers were affected by reading the PDQ in the patient's medical chart. Feedback was elicited from physicians, nurses, students (nursing, medicine, residents, interns), social workers, healthcare chaplains, and healthcare aides. One hundred thirty-seven healthcare providers provided feedback one or more times, yielding a total of 293 responses. Ninety percent indicated that they had learned some-thing new from the PDQ, 63% were emotionally affected by it, 63% reported an enhanced sense of connectedness to the patient, and 59% felt it influenced their empathy toward the patient, with just under half reporting that the PDQ enhanced their care for and respect toward the patient. Feedback included statements such as "I will be more aware of his pain levels and watch for signs and symptoms of discomfort" and "[the PDQ] accelerates the building trust part of the therapeutic relationship." It also appears that there were no differences in the ablity of the PDQ to influence healthcare providers when comparing responses gleaned from patients versus their family proxies. In other words, whether the patient or the family member was responsible for putting personhood on the clinical radar, the effect it had on healthcare providers was equally influential and potent.

There were some interesting differences in overall response to PDQ-elicited information among healthcare providers. For instance, students with little experience and physicians with more than 15 years of experience were most likely to be receptive to PDQs. It would thus appear that those more junior had the humility, while those more senior had the wisdom, to be open to hearing patients' stories. In general, female healthcare providers were significantly more likely to be responsive to information elicited by the PDQ. There was also significant variation across discipines, with physicians showing lowest responsiveness, followed by physician residents, then nurses, followed by social workers, chaplains, and healthcare aides, with nursing and medical students demonstrating highest responsiveness. Baseline characteristics such as empathy, social support, high job satisfaction, and a meaningful life were significantly associated with being responsive to PDQ-elicited information.

While the PDQ was largely developed and primarily examined in the context of terminal illness, it can readily be applied across the broad spectrum of medicine. Whether posed to a woman seeking prenatal care, a teenager asking for birth control, a young mother complaining of fatigue, or an elderly patient nearing end of life, conversations that ask about patients' stories are relevant across the entirety of the human life cycle. These conversations eliciting personhood result in patients feeling cared about and hence more satisfied with their care. Taking an interest in patients and what matters to them enhances trust, leading to personal disclosures that can inform medical decision-making, hence improving diagnostic accuracy and patient safety. The litmus test of PDQ endorsement was nearly every patient electing to have their PDQ summaries placed on their medical chart. This verifies that this information reflects how patients wish to be seen or wish their ill family member to be seen.

It is noteworthy that, in addition to the benefits accrued by patients and family members, the PDQ influenced healthcare providers, bolstering their sense of empathy, emotional connectedness, and overall understanding of the patient as a person. There was also an association between their receptiveness to the patient's story and overall capacity for empathy, finding meaning in their life, and overall job satisfaction. Because of the cross-sectional nature of these data we were unable to discern cause and effect. However, it is either the case that those who were most satisfied with their jobs were inclined to ask about the patient's story or thread or that eliciting patient's stories enhanced job satisfaction. The PDQ is not meant to replace more fulsome conversations with patients and families about their personal situation and what they deem important and wish to be known. However it does appear to provide a convenient starting point for further inquiry into matters about personhood. Clearly, dialogue that acknowledges patients as persons is critical to the delivery of dignity-conserving care. Cheryl Greaves, a clinical nurse specialist in medical oncology says, "I just hear the story and I can go there, it makes me feel what they're feeling. If I am interested in the story, I can get into their shoes and feel their pain. I have to go there. I have to be a part of them to understand what they are going through."

Conversations About Personhood and Families

Family members can serve an important role not only advocating on behalf of their loved ones, but also in reminding healthcare providers who this patient is or was as a person. Dr. Jeff Sisler is a family physician at CancerCare Manitoba with a special interest in medical oncology. He describes how a family member was instrumental in placing personhood on his clinical radar.

> The patient was well known in the hockey world, very well respected locally and nationally. He had an esophageal cancer, not a cancer where people generally do very well. I picked him up in the lung cancer clinic because of pain issues, after his first and second round of chemotherapy hadn't gone very well. I was working with a resident who had been involved in his care from the beginning, a year and a half ago, who described him as first presenting as a vigorous, fit, muscular, athletic, and dynamic guy. Over the course of his disease progression, he lost a hundred pounds, with all those terrible physical transformations that happen. So the guy in front of you isn't, at some level, really himself anymore. So when I met him I asked him to "tell me something about yourself, because I have never met you before and that would help me understand you a bit better." His wife responded by saying, "well, Jason's a pretty famous hockey player." It was as if she was telling me "you need to know this about my husband." She needed to do that because the man in front of me didn't look anything like the man she was describing. It turns out that he had

played briefly as a professional and coached at high levels as well. He remained connected with this important part of his life and the people in it, and I'd always check in on how that was going.

You might ask me, "Do I have time to get to know his hockey playing story?" My sense is that 90 seconds is enough to open that door, and you don't have to walk through it completely today. I don't think it takes a lot of time. The other thing is you sense how people blossom when you ask that question that allows them to say something about themselves, so they're glad to be acknowledged. There is a change in their demeanor. That's when everything changes and you sense that they are so desperately happy that someone is asking about their interests and passions and what gives their life meaning. "We've talked about your cancer, but tell me a little bit about yourself. What do you care about or are really interested in, so I can know you better as a person?" It just changes the nature of the relationship, from a technical one to one in which we share common interests. I'm interested in the Jets [hockey team] so it is just something about our common humanity. Emotionally, this feels like standing on holy ground, that you get to be with people in these very intimate times. He and his wife were such lovely people and he was young and his physical transformation was tragic. He died on Monday, and we last saw him in clinic on Friday. I just don't know how it would have been possible to care for this guy without knowing that he as a hockey player. Thinking about them is like having gone to a wonderful movie that has moved me and made me think, "How am I going to be in that moment when my time comes? How is my wife going to be, and am I going to have that kind of death?"

Conversations that Acknowledge Personhood and Intimate Care

Failure to see and acknowledge personhood can be especially devastating when the intimacies of care are onerous. Bodily excretions can assault the sensibilities of patients and healthcare providers alike. Carolyn Jardine describes how, as a nurse, she has done "some very unpleasant and hard, hard things. For instance, when a patient is super sick and they've soiled themselves. They may have just had GI surgery and they're soiling themselves with tons of blood and feces and its extremely scary, messy, and gross. A lot of people are so embarrassed and they can't imagine cleaning up that mess. And yet you do, with a smile and talking the whole time, maybe even a joke or a laugh at the end. And then you turn them carefully, remembering that they told you they had a really sore arm, and you made sure this was the first that you positioned when they were cleaned up. To do this work you need to consider how you would want to be treated in this situation, always be mindful of respect and think about them as a person. If they are talking, that allows you to connect with who they are as a person. Try distraction, or talk about something you know about them. Like, 'I see you have a picture. Was that drawn by your grand-child?' And so they start to talk about something personal, and they become a person in your mind. It's almost a religious act, like God put me here today because this person needed good care and I gave it to them."

While cleaning up someone who is soiled or emptying a bedpan are not often thought of as particularly important within the realm of healthcare, we need to consider how assaultive these can be on personhood and dig-nity. I recall speaking with an elderly gentleman in a personal care home who described the indignity of *having to go* in his diaper because healthcare aides routinely were not able to get to him on time. He recalled one occa-sion when he heard two healthcare aides arguing outside of his room door because neither wanted the unpleasant task of having to clean him up. More so than having to adjust to using a wheelchair or needing to accommodate to institutional time schedules around meals and visiting hours, this particular experience left him feeling dehumanized and emotionally eviscerated. When it comes to intimate dependencies, failure to acknowledge personhood can result in patients feeling reduced to their excrement. It takes exquisite skill and sensitivity to demonstrate that one always sees the person, no matter their bodily functions need attending.

Dr. Pam Orr recalls looking after a 28-year-old HIV patient who had devel-oped severe diarrhea due to *Cryptosporidium*. "This was back in the nineties when there was very little treatment for HIV. We tried to control his diarrhea but nothing seemed to work very well. He was having crippling diarrhea as a medical problem, and as a personal problem was struggling with the re-jection of his family. So he said to me, 'I don't want to die of diarrhea.' It still takes me aback a little bit because it makes me think that the diarrhea was an afront to his personal dignity. So I worked very hard in consultation with some other specialists to try to come up with some experimental methods to control his diarrhea, which we managed to get a handle on. In the end he died of PCP."

I recall my sister Ellen being in hospital on one of many occasions, crying because she had been having a particularly uncomfortable bout of diarrhea. I will never forget the healthcare aide who came into her room, sat on her bedside, and casually said, "I remember the last time I had diarrhea, my butt hurt for days." Ellen's crying immediately stopped and she smiled, instantly feeling reassured that we all have orifices, patients and healthcare providers alike, and that none of us is immune from times when orifices misbehave. It was a wonderful example of dignity in care, wherein the healthcare aide was able to see Ellen's vulnerability and assuage her sadness by affirming, in a very down to earth, authentic way, "I still see you and—guess what—you and I are not so different." This is reminiscent of Martin Buber's *I–Thou relationships*, which are described as real encounters, *when two people actively and authentically engage each other in the here and now and truly show up to one another.*[13] They are characterized by mutuality, directness, presentness, intensity, and ineffability. According to Buber, I–Thou relationships require *a bold leap into the experience of the other, while simultaneously being transparent, present, and accessible.* Buber saw the meeting between I and Thou as the most important feature of the human experience, one wherein we become fully human. On the other hand, *I–It relationships* are characterized by a lack of presence, *in which the other person is experienced as an object to be influenced or used—a means to an end*, and describe how we might act in response to an inanimate object. Buber called this deep participation with, and acceptance of, another's essential being "confirmation." He believed that *one's innate capacity to confirm others, and to be confirmed in one's own uniqueness by others, is the source of our humanity.*[14] When patients are feeling most under assault, when there is an inclination to objectify them based on their illness, their symptoms, or even their excrement—that is to see them as an *It*—Healthcare providers must strive toward entering into I-Thou relationships in which personhood, human dignity, and acknowledgment of our shared humanity can be sustained and confirmed.

References

1. Chochinov HM, Hack T, Hassard T, Kristjanson LJ, McClement S, Harlos M. Dignity in the terminally ill: A cross-sectional, cohort study. Lancet. 2002;360:2026–2030.
2. Chochinov HM, Kristjanson L, Hack T, Hassard T, McClement S, Harlos M. Dignity in the terminally ill: Revisited. J Palliat Med. 2006;9:666–672.
3. Chochinov HM. Dignity and the eye of the beholder. J Clin Oncol. 2004;22:1336–1340.
4. Schopenhauer A. *Essays and aphorisms*. Penguin Books; 1970.
5. Tolstoy L. *The death of Ivan Ilyich*. Bantam Classics; 1981.
6. Frazee C. *Dispatches from disabled country: Selected writings by Catherine Frazee*. In Press.
7. Chochinov HM. Seeing Ellen and The Platinum Rule. *JAMA Neurology*. In Press.
8. Swayden KJ, et al. Effect of sitting vs. standing on perception of provider time at bedside: A pilot study. Patient Educ Counsel. 2012:86:166–171
9. Herman RE, Williams KN. Elderspeak's influence on resistiveness to care: Focus on behavioral events. Am J Alzheimers Dis Other Demen. 2009;24:417–423
10. Levy B, Kunkel S. Longevity increased by positive self-perceptions of aging. J Person Soc Psychol. 2002;83(2):261–270.

11. Sinclair S, Beamer K, Hack TF, et al. Sympathy, empathy, and compassion: A grounded theory study of palliative care patients' understandings, experiences, and preferences. Palliat Med. 2017;31:437–447.
12. Farber S. Living every minute. J Pain Symptom Manage. 2015;49:796–800.
13. Chochinov HM, McClement S, Hack T, Thompson G, Dufault B, Harlos M. Eliciting personhood within clinical practice: Effects on patients, families and health care providers. J Pain Sympt Manage. 2015;17:1–28.
14. Martin M, Cowan EW. Remembering Martin Buber and the I-Thou in counseling. 2019. https://ct.counseling.org/2019/05/remembering-martin-buber-and-the-i-thou-in-counseling/

The Care of the Patient

The practice of medicine in its broadest sense includes the whole relationship of the physician with his patient. It is an art, based to an increasing extent on the medical sciences, but comprising much that still remains outside the realm of any science. The art of medicine and the science of medicine are not antagonistic but supplementary to each other. There is no more contradiction between the science of medicine and the art of medicine than between the science of aeronautics and the art of flying. Good practice presupposes an understanding of the sciences which contribute to the structure of modern medicine, but it is obvious that sound professional training should include a much broader equipment. . . .

The treatment of a disease may be entirely impersonal; the care of a patient must be completely personal. The significance of the intimate personal relationship between physician and patient cannot be too strongly emphasized, for in an extraordinarily large number of cases both diagnosis and treatment are directly dependent on it, and the failure of the young physician to establish this relationship accounts for much of his ineffectiveness in the care of patients. . . .

What is spoken of as a "clinical picture" is not just a photograph of a man sick in bed; it is an impressionistic painting of the patient surrounded by his home, his work, his relations, his friends, his joys, sorrows, hopes and fears. . . .

When a patient enters a hospital, one of the first things that commonly happens to him is that he loses his personal identity. He is generally referred to, not as Henry Jones, but as "that case of mitral stenosis in the second bed on the left." There are plenty of reasons why this is so, and the point is, in itself, relatively unimportant; but the trouble is that it leads, more or less directly, to the patient being treated as a case of mitral stenosis, and not as a sick man. The disease is treated, but Henry Jones, lying awake nights while he worries about his wife and children, represents a problem that is much more complex than the pathologic physiology of mitral stenosis, and he is apt to improve very slowly unless a discerning intern happens to discover why it is that even large doses of digitalis fail to slow his heart rate. Henry happens to have heart disease, but he is not disturbed so much by dyspnea as he is by anxiety for the future . . . but just because he is an interesting case he does not cease to be a human being with very human hopes and fears. . . .

There are moments, of course, in cases of serious illness when you will think solely of the disease and its treatment; but when the corner is turned and the immediate crisis is passed, you must give your attention to the patient. Disease in man is never exactly the same as disease in an experimental animal, for in man the disease at once affects and is affected by what we call the emotional life. Thus, the physician who attempts to take care of a patient while he neglects this factor is as unscientific as the investigator who neglects to control all the conditions that may affect his experiment.

The good physician knows his patients through and through, and his knowledge is bought dearly. Time, sympathy and understanding must be lavishly dispensed, but the reward is to be found in that personal bond which forms the greatest satisfaction of the practice of medicine. One of the essential qualities of the clinician is interest in humanity, for the secret of the care of the patient is in caring for the patient.

—Francis W. Peabody, MD
The care of the patient. *JAMA* 1927;88:877–882.

3
The Model of Optimal Therapeutic Communication

Thus far, the elements of dignity in care that have been covered include a detailed understanding of how patients respond to their changing health circumstances (Chapter 1) and how healthcare professionals indelibly shape every clinical encounter (Chapter 2). We are now ready to delve into the intricacies of optimal therapeutic communication, fundamental to achieving dignity in care.

Anyone who has studied medicine is well aware of the importance of learning about anatomical structures. Before being able to understand the functioning of a specific organ system, a thorough and detailed anatomical dissection is essential. While this process can be painstaking, it is foundational to understanding how form informs function. Without knowing the anatomical details and structures, it is simply not possible to fully grasp how the human body works. Communication, however, does not lend itself in the same way that physical structures do to anatomical dissection. And yet without some such attempt to disassemble the components of optimal therapeutic communication, we are unable to convey how this is best understood and achieved within the clinical setting. Although training guidelines for clinicians and therapists describe basic counseling competencies, there are few empirical models detailing the elements of effective, dignity-conserving communication. Such a model is critical, seeing it provides the closest approximation to anatomical dissection possible.

To begin this unique endeavor, we examined a body of communication knowledge gleaned from 78 experienced psychosocial oncology clinicians, from 24 health centers across Canada.[1] These clinicians were invited to participate in three focus groups each. In total, 29 focus groups were held over the course of 2 years, during which clinicians articulated therapeutic factors deemed most helpful in mitigating patients' psychosocial distress. Participants included 50 social workers, 8 physicians, 6 psychologists, 5 nurses, 5 spiritual care providers, and 4 other counselors. They had an average of 18 years of professional experience and 9 years experience in psychosocial oncology. On average, they saw 5 new patients per week within their healthcare setting, hospital inpatient/outpatient unit, or in hospice. The content of each focus group was summarized into major themes and reviewed with participants to confirm its accuracy. Upon completion of the focus groups, workshops were held in various centers to elicit participant feedback on an empirical model of optimal therapeutic effectiveness based on the qualitative analysis of focus group data. Upon completion of the model, 83% of respondents agreed or strongly agreed that it would enhance their ability to understand and address psychosocial distress with patients and clients, while 95% agreed or strongly agreed that the model would enhance their ability to teach others/students how to improve their ability to address psychosocial distress with patients and clients.

Model of Optimal Therapeutic Communication: Surface Dissection

A *surface dissection* identifies those components that are usually the first to be isolated during the process of disassembling anatomical structures. A similar surface dissection also applies to revealing the major components of optimal therapeutic communication. These surface elements included *therapeutic approaches, creation of a safe space,* and *personal growth and self-care* (see Figure 3.1).

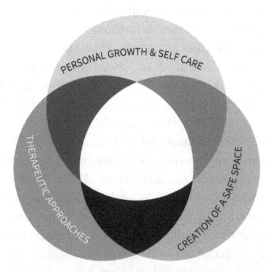

Figure 3.1 Surface dissection of model of optimal therapeutic effectiveness.

Therapeutic Approaches

This particular theme can be thought of as the therapeutic agenda one takes into any clinical encounter. "What am I here to do or trying to accomplish?" It might be any one of innumerable possibilities. Are you there to perform a physical examination or to take a history? Maybe you are scheduling an appointment or delivering food to their hospital room. Perhaps you are trying to get consent for a study or procedure? Maybe the agenda consists of meeting the patient for the first time and making introductions, or, on the more difficult end of the spectrum, perhaps you are there to deliver bad or difficult news. Being mindful of the agenda allows you to know what destination you are trying to reach. You may or may not be successful, but, like any destination, unless it is clearly identified, the likelihood of reaching that particular shore is profoundly diminished.

Because our study enrolled psychosocial clinicians, the agenda items they identified were largely within the realm of the emotional domains of patient experience. They included 16 themes (see Figure 3.2) that covered various tasks, strategies, or techniques that helped them to communicate with and support patients experiencing significant distress. These themes are tangible and teachable skill sets comprised of various clinical practices and approaches. They are not hierarchical nor are they mutually exclusive, and their presence is entirely dependent on the nature of the clinical encounter. For example, a highly distressed or emotional patient may respond to clinicians who help them *to clarify and name their sources of distress* along with *problem-solving*. On the other hand, patients who are pensive or reticent to talk about their turmoil may respond to therapeutic approaches comprised of *probing for feelings underlying events and circumstances* or *acknowledging spiritual distress*.

Therapeutic approaches are usually chartable activities or events, denoting what was done or accomplished during the course of a given clinical encounter. *The procedure was explained. Consent was obtained. The patient's questions were answered. The patient's concerns were identified and named. The patient's problem with pain/depression/anxiety was addressed.*

Sometimes the therapeutic agenda may be very specific, such as explaining a procedure, providing an intervention, or offering a diagnosis or prognosis. At other times it may be more vague, such as checking in to see how the patient is doing or simply dropping in to demonstrate that we are still involved, available, and attentive. Having some clarity on the therapeutic approach or agenda is akin to knowing where you are heading. When you know where you are going, you are much more likely to get there.

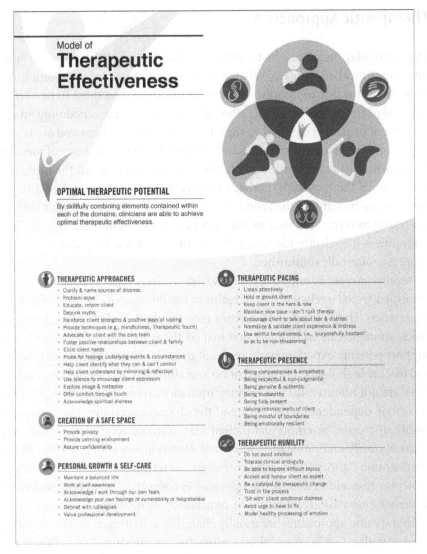

Figure 3.2 Model of therapeutic effectiveness.[1]

Creating a Safe Space

> Privacy is a privilege not granted to the aged or the young.
> — **Margaret Laurence,** *The Stone Angel*

This particular domain is comprised of three themes: *provide privacy, provide a calming environment,* and *assure confidentiality.* This domain refers to the therapeutic setting or milieu wherein the patient feels safe and secure.

It is within theses settings that patients are most likely to reveal what is really on their minds. Jill Taylor-Brown reminds us that, "in order for someone to tell you what is bothering them, what's concerning them the most, what symptoms they are having, they need to feel safe, and in order to feel safe with you and to trust you and to be able to tell you what is really gong on, they need to feel that you are seeing all of them." Creating a safe space fosters a setting wherein clinicians do their best to convey to patients that *this is their exclusive time: I'm here to see you and only you.* Although an office or meeting room may be the ideal, sometimes a drawn curtain or even physical proximity can be used to great effect to create a sense of intimacy and privacy.

Even if a therapeutic approach is executed perfectly, failure to *create a safe space* will undermine and taint its integrity, leading patients to feel more vulnerable, withdrawn, or even emotionally assaulted. Imagine a physical examination in which the door to the patient's room is not fully closed or a curtain between the patient's bed and the one next to it is left partially askew. In these circumstances patients are bound to feel embarrassed or that their basic right to privacy and preserved modesty have been violated. To be cavalier about *creating a safe space* conveys the message that those things don't matter, closely approximating the logical conclusion that "you don't matter, betraying your privacy and breaking of your confidence are inconsequential."

Bridget Johnson is a Communication Clerk at CancerCare Manitoba. She recalled a woman who had actually been a mentor of hers through high school and who was now a patient being provided care for a gynecological malignancy. "She was put in a gown in a room and then left there for an hour. She came out so distressed and said, "How dare they do this to me. This is so wrong. I'm not comfortable sitting like this." Patients are particularly vulnerable, and this patient's sense of her privacy being violated was, while unintentional, profound. Of course healthcare providers don't commit these transgressions on purpose, but more often, these considerations simply fall off their radar.

So you are about to enter into a patient's hospital room. He is a 67-year-old farmer from rural Manitoba. He is a husband, father, and grandfather, known within his community to be a Mr. Fix-it. He came to medical attention a few weeks ago because one day, while fixing some farm equipment, he spat-up some blood. He has had various blood tests and scans as part of his workup, but a few days ago was admitted to the hospital with increasing weakness and shortness of breath. His biopsy results, confirming he has small cell lung cancer, have yet to be discussed with him. The clinical task is clear. He needs to be given this information. But how can this life-changing conversation take place in a way that is mindful of *creating a safe space* in which this diagnosis can be shared? Is there a family member with him or is he alone? Is the room door shut? Is the curtain drawn? Is there relative quiet so all parties can be heard? Knowing the clinical task that needs to be accomplished, the sharing of information and creating a safe space for this painful disclosure constitute the first two elements of our surface dissection.

Personal Growth and Self-Care

The third element identified in the surface dissection of this body of communication knowledge is a domain labeled *personal growth and self-care* (see Figures 3.1 and 3.2). This is comprised of six themes including: *maintaining a balanced life, working at self-awareness, acknowledging/working through one's own fears, acknowledging one's own feelings of vulnerability or helplessness, debriefing with colleagues*, and *valuing professional development*. These themes refer to clinicians' internal psyche and personal sense of well-being, which shape their responses within the therapeutic encounter along with ways in which those can be fostered and nurtured, such as seeking out support from colleagues, valuing professional development, and maintaining a balance between personal and professional life. As Parker Palmer has said, in our interaction with another person what matters most is not only what we do, how we do it, or why we do what we do, but who we bring to each interaction.[2] Regarding the latter, Dr. Gingerich says, "you need to be aware of and engaged with the patient, but you also need to be aware of yourself, and make sure that there are professional boundaries and that you are taking care of yourself." The domain of personal growth and self-care underscores that who you are as a person—your personality, your outlook, your demeanor—is critical in shaping every clinical encounter. As healthcare professionals, we bring the entirety of who we are to the bedside or outpatient clinic, which means we must be mindful of the profound influence our personality, sense of well-being, and disposition will have on the way we interact with patients.

To foster personal growth and promote self-care, healthcare providers need to be mindful that the challenges they face are not easily compartmentalized and that debriefing is critical. Take the case of a 14-year-old girl described by Dr. Mike Harlos as dying of cancer, who has shown a big change in the last 24 hours, "actually since 5 o'clock this morning. There was sudden pain, which is now under control, but it looks like time is down to a day or two. While the bedside nurse is telling me all that has gone on and how she got on top of things, I ask her how she is doing with this. People don't ask bedside nurses 'How are you doing with this?' And she's doing okay, but she's known this girl since she was diagnosed a couple of years ago." This kind of debriefing and checking in is critical. "It's not just all business and technical. So you ask 'Are you doing ok?' and you see that she is committed to see that this girl will be comfortable when she dies. She has made that promise to herself and to the family." He also says that people need to be self-aware.

> I guess it's about mindfulness, being self-aware about how things are affecting you, anticipating that this is going to be tough. I better be aware of what it feels like in that room. And like a surfer, finding a balance is moment by moment, in fact it's second by second. I think you need to be close enough that it's a little raw. It's like standing next to a heat source or fire, you've got to find a distance that is safe but still effective. . . . It's not like you decide to take this approach and are good for your career, its more like deciding to lose 30 pounds. It's not a one-time decision: you have to be mindful every time you have the option of taking the stairs or not, or eating that dessert or not. I remember talking with a friend who is an Orthodox Jew and asking him to describe his spiritual practice, and he said that he is always mindful of his faith. For him, like the person losing weight, there is a thread of consciousness that weaves into the tapestry of every waking moment. So in our work there is this kind of perpetual awareness. It's not easy and there is no way that I'm unaffected by what I see when I walk into that room. I don't think you can be an effective palliative care doctor, in fact be an effective human being, unless you attend to the needs of others. But I've learned over 20 years where and how to package it, what you need to take ownership of, and what you can't take ownership of.
>
> Boundaries can also become blurred when healthcare providers fall into the seduction of "I'm so special." There's a real danger in that. Patients and families start telling you how special you are, your colleagues sometimes do, and you start believing it and that's where things start to unravel. You start to think that "I am special," no one else can do this like I can. You start giving your home phone numbers and cell numbers, or saying "wait until I'm back on service and then we'll deal with that." You end up trying to be the one and all for their care needs, independent of your colleagues and the system, and it becomes impossible to meet all of their needs. So when people are becoming intensely involved and not relying on colleagues and the system, I would argue they are actually doing a disservice to that patient and family. And we see this all the time.

Debriefing and checking in is a way of ensuring that healthcare providers are attending to the psychological and spiritual demands of their jobs. Healthcare providers may carry these feeling into their personal lives in the same way that baggage from our personal life can easily spill over into our professional life. The end of a work day does not mean that work-related thoughts won't linger. In reflecting on things that *keep me up at night*, Dr. Michael West shared what happens when anticipating a particularly complicated case. "You know that you have the skills, the technology, and the capacity to do this, the stakes are high, but you don't have a choice. That is so often the case in neurosurgery. Say you have a tumor in the third ventricle and it is going to be extremely difficult to approach it and get it out without causing a problem, never mind the risk of the patient dying. That makes me lose sleep. You have studied the images and considered approaches, and you find yourself, nights before, waking up and thinking about it because of the concern about inflicting damage on someone. It is helpful to plan ahead for sure and to plan and figure out what you are going to do, but it is not helpful to be waking up at night and worrying about it."

He also addresses self-awareness in observing that "as you get older, although you are more experienced, there are some things that get more difficult emotionally, because you are getting more into a position where you should be the person that is sick and not the healing individual looking after patients. You have been through all of these stages of life and you have a better understanding of what the challenges are when you are 20, when you are 30, when you are 40. You are just getting married, you are just starting a family. Now you are just starting a job. You have been through all of that yourself, so it gives you a totally different understanding. Just the concept of a loving relationship with a spouse, with a family. You know what that is now, in a way you didn't when you were younger. This informs you but can also make it harder, because these people have these tremendous challenges. They don't have the chance to really savor life, and they are not going to have a chance to complete it, or they will complete it with a deficit. So there is a sense of inequity, that you have passed those stages and you are home free and these people are going to have to struggle with it. And it makes me wonder, 'How have I managed to get to this age and avoided all of this?'"

Not surprisingly, the domain of personal growth and self-care contains themes that shape our demeanor and implicate our fears, our feelings of vulnerability, helplessness, and need for self-care in establishing a sustainable work-life balance. Dr. West says that "to be a neurosurgeon, you have to have stamina so you have to do something to keep yourself physically healthy. In the past, I have been a runner and that is one of those things where you can get out and really get that endorphin rush, which makes you feel good and gives you time to think. . . . I am very fortunate that I have a supportive wife and family. I missed many birthday parties and soccer games because I was at the hospital. They put up with me when I was busy, but now they are starting to tell me the stories of how they felt at those times."

In reflecting on the challenges of finding a home-work-life balance, Dr. Robert Lotocki says, "Not to sound selfish, but you need to sometimes get out of the hospital. You can't look after cancer 24/7 and still maintain a social, personal life outside of the institution. But even then your patients still come with you. If you are sitting and watching a hockey game, you find yourself thinking about patients and forgetting about the hockey game that is on the ice. So in that way you never leave it. It's not a 9-to-5 job. When 5 o'clock comes along, you take some of the work home with you. It is the mental work that comes with you. You may have a person that you are managing and you are thinking, 'Am I doing the right thing for this person at this time?' You have seen them and have already set them up. But they might be having a tough time with their disease. It doesn't stop at 5 o'clock. It continues when you go home. I don't talk to my wife about cases. I just don't think she needs that hassle. But you are dealing with human beings and you are a human being. You don't stop just because you left work. Sometimes you wonder how you got home. You know you have driven the car and it has gone from CancerCare to home, and I think, 'How did I get here?'"

Self-awareness, or lack thereof, can profoundly shape the clinical encounter. Many years ago I was asked to see a woman referred by her nurse, who described her patient as demanding and uncooperative. As I recall the patient was in her early 40s, had three children between the ages of 10 and 15 years old, and had a diagnosis of acute myeloid leukemia. She struck me as bright, insightful, and, as far as I could determine, cooperative with her care. Her primary struggle was coming to terms with a dire prognosis and anticipating how her children would cope in the event of her death. As I shared my impressions with her nurse, who also happened to be in her early 40s, it emerged that, like her patient, she, too, was the mother of three young children. In the course of our discussion, it soon became apparent that the identification she felt with the patient contributed to her negative perceptions and accounted for the difficulties that had resulted in my being consulted. The ability to acknowledge her own sense of vulnerability and helplessness fostered a healthier therapeutic connection, allowing her to provide the care, personal insight, and support this patient desperately craved. As Sue Bates said, we need to be mindful that we are not so very different than our patients. "It could be your mom, it could be your dad, it could be a brother or sister, it could be the guy next door; so knowing that, you need to make the time to listen, so the patient and family feel that they have been heard and their worries have been listened to."

Besides being certain of the clinical agenda (therapeutic approaches) and creating a safe space, the domain of personal growth and self-awareness underscores that clinicians invariably bring elements of themselves into the clinical encounter that influence their degree of therapeutic effectiveness. Returning to the gentleman to whom we were about to reveal a diagnosis of small cell lung cancer—now that we are clear about the clinical task at hand and have created a safe space for this encounter to occur, such as closing the door, drawing a curtain, sitting down, and moving close enough so the patient won't have to strain to hear—we need to be mindful of those aspects of our-selves that we bring into the clinical encounter. If we fail to be aware that this is a life-altering conversation, if our own need to protect ourselves from the pa-thos of this encounter means complete disavowal of its emotional resonance, it is almost certain that we will be perceived as cold and unfeeling, no matter how clinically accurate our information about small cell lung cancer may be. Perhaps the patient reminds us of ourselves, or a father, grandfather, spouse, brother, or neighbor. The fact that he is a handyman and farmer may trigger other associations which will humanize him in a way that makes him more than the embodiment of his malignancy. Recognition and acknowledgment of these connections are meant to invoke compassion and an appreciation for the human drama that is unfolding concurrent with the wayward physiolog-ical happenings. Although you cannot change the facts of his medical condi-tion and prognosis, you can change his perception of whether you genuinely care about him and see him beyond the radiologic shadow cast by his tumor. Such recognition is not meant to emotionally unhinge or overwhelm you, but nor should it underwhelm you. Awareness of who he is as a person is meant to invoke responses based on who you are, thereby informing your tone of care. "Is this a good time for an important conversion? I'm afraid the news isn't what we hoped it would be. I wish I didn't have to tell you this. I can only im-agine how disappointing this must be for you and your family. When you've had time to absorb this and talk it over with your family, I'd like to meet with you again, so I can answer your questions and we can begin to plan next steps for your care." You will find your own words and they will be appropriate so long as they are delivered from the vantagepoint of genuine caring and con-cern. *Patients may forget what you say or do, but they will long remember how you make them feel.* Jill Taylor-Brown says that "people will describe how they were told that the chemo was no longer working, that there is no other chemo that they think will be effective, that the cancer is progressing. That really dif-ficult conversation that we are moving toward end of life, that transition con-versation. Every single time that a patient has said to me that I could tell that it was really hard for the doctor to tell me this, they felt good about that. They could see humanness in the healthcare provider, that they saw them as a real human being that was important to them."

A social worker who participated in the communication dissection research study arrived late one day for our regularly scheduled focus group. She explained that she had been delayed, having to await a patient whose signature she required. Using the model, we unpacked this encounter as follows. The therapeutic task was clear: she required a signature from the patient on a long-term disability form. She had asked to meet the patient at her office, allowing for maximum confidentiality and privacy, thereby creating a safe space. Why, I asked, had she simply not asked someone else to get his signature? A ward clerk or administrative assistant could just as easily have retrieved that, allowing this social worker to make our research focus group on time. She explained that this would not have been suitable, and while, it may have accomplished the designated task, it would have fallen far short of *optimal therapeutic efficacy*. As it turned out, the patient had an advanced malignancy and had gone through rounds of chemotherapy and radiation over the course of several years. Despite knowing he was running out of curative options, he had doggedly tried to maintain his work routine. With further disease progression, he now faced having to relinquish employment permanently. The social worker understood that, for this patient, working was closely aligned with his sense of personal identity. Not working raised the question of not only "What will I do?" but more pointedly, "Who will I be?" While recognizing this dynamic made this social worker more emotionally vulnerable, it also helped her recognize exactly what this man needed when handing over these forms for his signature: recognition of this watershed moment and the tremendous emotional weight it carried. Such recognition, even if only conveyed through the tone of care, perhaps a gentle touch, a kind word ("I can only imagine how hard this must be for you") helped the social worker ensure this encounter was optimally therapeutically effective.

Model of Optimal Therapeutic Communication: Deeper Dissection

Having completed the surface dissection of this body of communication knowledge, we proceeded to cut deeper into the data. As illustrated in the model (see Figure 3.3), there are three places where the primary domains overlap one another. This means that we identified themes that did not exclusively fit into one of the three primary domains but rather seemed to overlap or straddle two domains. Understanding these areas of overlap, or hybrid domains, offers additional insight into achieving optimal therapeutic efficacy.

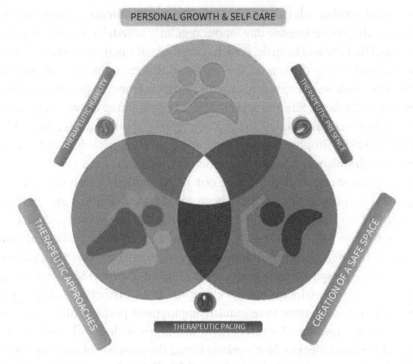

Figure 3.3 Primary domains: Model of therapeutic effectiveness.

Therapeutic Pacing

Seven themes overlapped between *therapeutic approaches* and *creating a safe space*. Collectively these themes describe and are labeled *therapeutic pacing*. Each of these themes refers to a therapeutic strategy that concurrently implicates the intensity or flow of the therapeutic process, hence creating a safe space. These include:

- Listening attentively
- Holding or grounding the patient
- Keeping the patient in the here and now
- Using skillful tentativeness (i.e., being purposefully hesitant to be nonthreatening)
- Maintaining a slow pace (i.e., not rushing the therapy)
- Encouraging the client to talk about their fear and distress
- Normalizing and validating the patient's experience and distress

Too slow a pace, which deals only with *here-now* issues and avoids exploring deeper content, can leave patients feeling frustrated or psychologically stuck.

On the other hand, a therapeutic pace that is too confrontational or emotionally evocative can cause patients to feel overwrought and overwhelmed. Therapeutic pacing can be thought of, metaphorically, as the accelerator within the communication apparatus. There are times when the therapeutic task is to draw back on the accelerator, establishing a pace that is nonconfrontative and protects patients from the onslaught of emotional flooding. One research participant shared an incident in which she had been called "stat" to the oncology clinic. She came upon a scene wherein the patient, a highly distraught woman, was crouched on the floor of an examination room crying inconsolably. She had just been given the dire news that her prognosis was much worse than she had expected. The therapeutic task in this instance was all about creating a safe space, which could only be accomplished by pacing consisting of a complete withdrawal from the metaphorical accelerator. This was not a time to encourage the patient to talk about her fears and distress (e.g., "What was it like to hear words like terminal or palliative?") but rather to engage techniques that reference themes such as *holding or grounding the patient, keeping the patient in the here and now, maintaining a slow pace*, and *normalizing and validating the patient's experience and distress*. In this instance, the social worker shut the clinic room door, creating a safe space, and sat down on the floor beside her, gently took her hand, and said, "all you need to do right now is just breathe."

Another way to control the pace in a fashion that is nonthreatening is to use skillful hesitancy or tentativeness. This approach is comprised of posing open-ended questions in which you use your own ostensible lack of understanding to elicit patient engagement and feedback. For example, the patient refusing analgesia despite her obvious discomfort. Rather than telling her, yet again, her options for pain relief, you enlist her input by asking her to help you understand why she is making this seemingly illogical choice: "I'm struggling here. Can you help me understand why you don't want to take these pain medications?" I recall one such case of a woman who responded by disclosing that her mother had died a horrible death and that, just prior to dying, had been placed on morphine. For her, accepting opioids somehow meant that her final illness would follow her mother's course. This technique can also be invaluable when the patient poses a question that pushes you off balance: "How long have I got to live?" or "If my dad was a dog, you would have put him down by now." Dr. Harlos says that this is akin to when a boxer gets hit in the head. "They will move into a well-practiced framework, when for about 5 or 10 seconds they cover-up, fall against the ropes, try to gather their wits about them, and then re-engage. When we are asked questions that have thrown us off balance, you need a framework that has several steps. One is to acknowledge the question and normalize it. 'That is a really good question,' or 'that is an important comment. I have heard a lot of people say that kind of thing.' This is an acknowledgment, you have normalized it and already made a connection. Next you say, 'Can you help me understand what's making you ask that today?' That's where you find out what the agenda is. That simple exploration has been responsible for a few weddings on the palliative care unit because while the patient's question was 'Am I dying, and how long have I got?' the underlying issue revealed was that his daughter is getting married in 3 months and he wants to walk her down the aisle and he won't be around even a month from now. So now we understand his agenda, can figure out what to do, move up the wedding, and have it on the unit."

Dr. Harlos describes another important step in this framework, comprised of saying to the patient, "When people ask this question, they've often thought a lot about it, because it's a thoughtful question, and they often have some idea of the answer themeselves. 'I'm wondering, if your friend came in and asked you that same question, tell me what you would say to them?' This is really a way of saying, 'tell me what your understanding is about things and what you expect.'"

Achieving optimal therapeutic pacing is akin to what Dr. Harlos describes as *titrating communication*. "In managing symptoms with a drug", he says, "you are titrating a drug to a desired outcome or effect. You do that by looking up the starting dose of a drug, you often tend to start conservative, and then you titrate to observe the effect. In communication, you are titrating information in order to convey a message, and your outcome is that the message is conveyed. So how do you look up a starting dose? Well, you do that by exploring the knowledge and understanding that the patient already has about the issue. You look in the chart and perhaps you see that the patient has been told about his diagnosis, he's been told that we are going to come see him, and maybe that he's decided he wants comfort-focused care. So that helps judge his 'starting dose'—the nature of the beginning of the dialogue. If we are talking about a child, again, you would look in the chart, talk to the clinical team and the parents, asking them to tell you about what your child understands, and that informs the starting dose of information. When I walk into the room, I would say for example, 'I'm Dr. Harlos and I'm with the team that helps with pain and other symptoms when people have serious illness.' Words like *palliative care* are a pretty hefty starting dose of information. By asking 'Can you tell me what your understanding is about what's happening, and what people have told you?' I can gauge how to begin the conversation— how tentative to be, what pace of information sharing might be best. This is how I explore the starting dose. For the patient who replies with 'I don't know anything about what's going on—nobody tells me anything' there will be a different approach than for the one who answers 'Well, they told me things are really bad and that I might have only a week or two.' "

There are times when the therapeutic pacing requires a more emotionally evocative stance, engaging themes such as *encouraging the patient to talk about their fear and distress* or invoking a technique of purposeful hesitancy. "I'm not sure I understand? When you say you've had enough, how am I to understand that?" For example, there may be instances where the patient is having a hard time talking about their distress or anguish or has chosen to largely not address their anxieties and fears. Gentle pressure on the communication acelerator may lead to a question such as, "Can we talk about how you are feeling? Can you tell me where your mind takes you to in the quiet of the night?" Therapeutic pacing must be tailored to suit the patient's specific needs and should be adjusted, moment to moment, within the therapeutic encounter. Dr. Harlos points out that, "sometimes, externally, people may not be acknowledging what's going on, maybe they're not crying as much as people think they should be, or they are not saying the words *'death and dying,'* or they are talking about all of them going to the lake next summer."

This can be concerning to the healthcare team, and the families may be described with terms such as "They don't get it." You can imagine that the healthcare team might be in the *we get it room*, where the gravity of the situation is understood, while the patient and/or family might be in the *we don't get it room*, where there does not appear to be a recognition or acknowledgment of the severity of the condition. I would argue there is a foyer, a common room between them which I would call the *scary what-if room*. The key to understanding the *scary what-if room* is that any of us in a frightening or threatening situation can think of *scary what-ifs*. You have an exam tomorrow morning, you're going to court, you're up the night before, going "What-if, what-if I get asked the wrong question? What if I totally bomb? What if my test tomorrow shows I actually do have something really bad?" All of those *what-ifs*. So the family, say in the ICU, that seems not to be getting it, you can bet are having sleepless nights and scary *what-ifs*. So I might say, "I know you're hoping we can turn this around and I need you to understand that everything we're doing is toward that goal, and none of the things we're suggesting for comfort is threatening that goal. But in my experience, families in this situation, in the dark hours of the night might find that their mind wanders to the scary 'what-if' places, and I'm wondering if that's the case for you?" Almost always they will say, "yeah, of course I do," and then I say to them, "Is that something we can talk about—consider a plan in case a what-if scenario develops—and then wrap it up and put it in a corner?" Not necessarily deal with it but acknowledge it and talk about it, so we have a way of approaching them. Sometimes I'll say, "my guess is you have got a fire extinguisher in your kitchen. You're not planning a fire, you're not hoping for a fire, but you have acknowledged the scary 'what-if' and bought it, and put it away in the corner. That's what this conversation is like. It doesn't mean that we're embracing the fact that you or your family member might die, or that we are hoping for anything other than a complete recovery." The scary *what-if* room is a useful idea, because there are very few people in a horrible situation that don't have these thoughts.

Sometimes attentiveness to pacing means taking the necessary time to complete a therapeutic task, such as the retrieval or conveyance of information, while allowing the necessary time for patients' and families' emotional processing. Dr. Gingrich recounted the case of an elderly gentleman, "who had been deteriorating and the family had a lot of anxiety around this issue. There had been lots of calls coming into the cancer centre about what to do with him. So I decided that I would meet them to talk about the symptoms that he was having and see where things were at. Through the conversation it became clear that he was deteriorating to the point that we wouldn't be able to start chemotherapy, which had been the plan all the way along. Transitioning to palliative care would be most appropriate. I remember purposefully making the point to try and take my time, answer their questions, and not rush it at all. By the end of the conversation, we had given them bad news, telling them what it meant, news they had never heard before, or news that hadn't previously registered. We came to the conclusion that we should really transition to palliative care and supportive care and set things up for him at home for the time that he had left. It was a very important outcome, given where things had been when they came in, because there was a lot of anxiety and they didn't really have a game plan or know where they were going. By the end, we had that set up. And it didn't take that long for him to pass away, but I remember them telling me how much they appreciated that meeting. It was a long interaction, but reflecting back on it and hearing how much it meant to their family, it was very powerful."

Delivering bad news is a time when one needs to pay particular attention to pacing. Finding out what patients already know and asking about what they would like to know now is an important part of setting the stage for these conversations. Dr. Lotocki recalls a colleague who struggled with this difficult clinical task. "She did not do it very well. She did not personalize it. It was *talk fast and just get the information out.* That is not what a person needs when they are getting bad news. They need to hear it at their speed. The key thing is also the ablity to listen and not just put the information on the table. But being open to all of their questions and giving them time to digest what they've been told before jumping to the next piece of information. So be sure to listen and do not interrupt. Just let the patient do the talking. And get comfortable using words like 'I don't know' rather than having all the answers when there are no right answers to be had." Also be sure to clarify what you are being asked. Dr. Harlos says, "I assume when someone says 'How long have I got?' I assume it means how long am I going to live, until one fellow said to me, 'Whoa, I think you're telling me when I'm going to die. I just want to know when I'm getting out of the hospital.' I've learned to clarify the question by asking 'Are you wondering how long you might have to live?' And the phrase 'how long you might have to live' can be easier to say and hear than 'when you think they will die.' It's really like the difference between 'this isn't survivable' versus 'you're going to die no matter what we do'—they may both accurately reflect the reality of the situation, but one feels more gentle."

Sometimes delivering bad news requires teamwork; some members of the team may be more skilled or have more time available than others or may be more suited to the unique scenario at hand due to language or cultural considerations. As Dr. Harlos outlines, "you're on the medicine service and you've got to go tell Mr. Jones that the reason he's come in and is tired and has weakness on his left side is that you've figured out he's got metastatic lung cancer with two brain mets, and the trouble is you've got 30 other patients to see that day. There is no way you can spend anything more than a few minutes at the bedside, during which you tell him we know what's going on, here are the results, and we're going to get oncology, radiation oncology, and see what they have to say. The trouble is that this poor gentleman is devastated. You haven't asked him how this is going to impact his family, if he wants us to speak with them, and how he's going to deal with this. So I would talk to the social worker on our program and say we are about to go in with Mr. Jones. Can you come in with us and, after we leave, hang back as we leave and say, 'That was tough news. Tell me what that was like.' So you work as a team."

Sometimes therapeutic pacing can be thwarted by the antithesis of attentive listening and encouraging the patient to talk about their concerns and fears. Caroline Jardine recalled working with a doctor "who could be patronizing and not listen, usually to female patients anxious that they might have a recurrence. This male doctor would tap the patient on the head and say, 'it's okay, don't worry about it.' When an older man taps you on the head and says 'its okay, don't worry about it,' it's demeaning and makes you feel like 'I'm not six years old and you're not my father,' and makes you feel like what you've said is silly, when it's not silly at all. Instead you need someone to explain why they are so confident that everything is going to be okay, instead of just saying 'don't worry.'"

And while clinicians often worry about how much time therapeutic communication can take, a therapeutic connection can quickly be established with a kind word, an empathic glance, a spontaneous gesture. Dr. Harlos insists that, "it really does not take a lot of time." He explains that, "you can usually tell in the first few seconds of interaction with someone, such as a physician, a store clerk, or a server in a restaurant, whether you're connecting. Eye contact, body language or posture, a look or a touch, all can quickly convey attentiveness and connection. A physician might simply say 'How's it going, tell me what you're concerned or worried about?'; this in fact will save time. When people have complaints and concerns about their interactions with physicians, communication problems are a common thread seen—either as the main issue or as a major contributing factor. Trying to repair damaged trust after the fact or to address such concerns through formal processes such as the professional regulatory body or litigation is much more time-consuming than spending a few moments attending to those needs in the moment. Similarly, when you go to a restaurant you might have a server who is engaged and energetic and connects to you, or alternatively might be inattentive, disengaged, and seems apathetic about your experience. There's no difference in the time it takes, but the tips will sure be very different."

After his initial diagnosis of colon cancer, Tom Roche shared this anecdote: "I was waiting to get a CT scan, and the chap who'd done the colonoscopy saw me in the waiting room and came over and just put his hand on my shoulder and said, 'You're going to be fine.' And that was huge. It took 30 seconds, but for me, that made a tremendous difference. At that particular time I was very anxious and there was a lot of uncertainty and I didn't know what might happen. And it took 30 seconds, but the message was really very powerful and very helpful for me, even though I never saw him again. A whole-person approach doesn't have to be sitting down with somebody for an hour; it can just be the way someone looks at you, or listens for a minute or two. This sort of gentle reassurance may take a few seconds but it can make a big difference."

As Tom attests, the tone of care can transform even the briefest of interactions into a positive encounter. "Patients understand that you may only have 10 or 15 minutes for a session, but it's what happens in those moments that matters. Sit down, be attentive, be present and open, listen to their concerns, and respond as best you can. That can happen very quickly, say hello, shake hands, smile, invite people in, this doesn't take long to do." It is also the fact that clinicians who try to run away from patient and family questions spend their careers feeling chased.

Therapeutic Presence

Eight themes reside at the interface between *creating a safe space* and *personal growth and self-care*. These are themes wherein personal qualities and attributes of the clinician directly contribute to and are indivisible from the sense of safety or security that patients experience as part of the therapeutic milieu. Collectively these themes were labeled *therapeutic presence* and markedly shape the tone of care. They speak to qualities that clinicians can invoke, or embody, that create a safe space for the therapeutic encounter to occur. They include:

- Being compassionate and empathetic
- Being respectful and nonjudgmental
- Being genuine and authentic
- Being trustworthy
- Being fully present
- Being mindful of boundaries
- Being emotionally resilient
- Valuing the intrinsic worth of the patient

Each of these requires clinicians to draw on deeply held personal qualities which operate in the service of making patients feel valued, affirmed, and understood. Failure to evince these qualities can undermine patients' feeling of safety and comfort, hence threatening optimal therapeutic effectiveness. For example, the clinician who is not *fully present*, distracted by their telephone or pager or other competing interests, can cause patients to feel unworthy of their undivided attention. When attentiveness is sporadic or easily diverted, patients can easily conclude that their condition, worries, or anguish are not being fully appreciated or understood. The healthcare system meant to look after them will no longer feel like a safe place wherein healing and safety can be sought. Failure to *value the intrinsic worth of the patient* can lead people to feel unimportant or devalued. This can be especially true for patients with chronic illnesses, disabilities, or life-limiting conditions. Catherine Frazee, a preeminent disability rights advocate who lives with spinal muscular atrophy describes how healthcare provider disposition and perspective can shape the therapeutic encounter: "Having to wear diapers and drooling are highly stigmatized departures from what is expected of adult bodies. Those of us who deviate from these norms experience social shame and stigma that erodes resilience and increases vulnerably. The more deeply these stigmatized accounts are embedded in our discourse and social policy, the more deeply virulent social prejudice takes hold within our culture. . . . What assurance can we offer that the physician who treats these adults at end of life will not stand at their bedside with horror, or revulsion, in his heart?"[3] Seeing patients through a lens of therapeutic nihilism and bias can lead to the conclusion that nothing is worth trying and certain lives are not worth preserving. One can also easily imagine a clinician *letting nature takes its course* as a solution for a clinical situation they could fathom neither themselves nor those they love being able to bear. Consistent with the Golden Rule, they might infer that "I wouldn't want to live this way" leading to *distorted compassion*—that is, compassion based on tainted or inaccurate perceptions of suffering, leading to ostensibly well-intended advice, actions, or inactions that may be completely at odds with what the patient really wants. Rather than feeling that they have been heard, distorted compassion can result in patients feeling devalued and further demoralized at the very hands of those who are meant to help. In those instances, a Platinum Standard—*do unto patients as they would want done unto themselves*—is required (see Chapter 2).

While we need to be emotionally attuned to our patients lived experience, we cannot take ownership of their plight. Emotional attunement brings us close enough to appreciate their circumstances, while keeping us distant enough to maintain sound clinical objectivity and judgment. This is a continuous negotiation, which harkens back to Dr. Harlos's surfer metaphor. Being too far back from the wave is the equivalent of emotional disconnectedness. Being *too close*, on the other hand, can be experienced as a failure to be emotionally resilient, which can lead patients to withhold emotionally evocative material as a means of protecting the clinician who has become too emotionally involved and fragile.

Finding the optimal empathic distance is no easy task and is part of maintaining professional boundaries. As Dr. Harlos says, "it's important as a physician dealing with a clinical situation to be aware of what you *own* (are responsible to address and attend to and are accountable for) and what you cannot own—which you simply have no control over. In the context of palliative and end-of-life care, the physician must *own* being clinically capable, managing pain and other symptoms, being a compassionate and effective communicator, ensuring there are supports available for patient and family needs (such as after-hours calls and possible visits), working professionally with healthcare colleagues, etc.—this is already a lot and is not comprehensive. However, there are elements of the end-of-life experience that are impactful and burdensome, but which a physician cannot *own*. Trying to do so may contribute to exhaustion and burnout. These include the sadness and unfairness of the circumstances and the very fact of the diagnosis. You can be supportive for such issues and engage available colleagues and resources as possible, but you can't make dying not sad or not unfair."

Each of the themes subsumed in the domain of therapeutic presence indicates ways in which the clinician draws on deeply held personal qualities that are invoked in the service of maintaining safety, over and above maintaining privacy, confidentiality, and providing a calm environment. Even when patients are seen in the hurly-burly of a busy ward or outpatient clinic, therapeutic presence can establish a milieu wherein patients feels safe, acknowledged, and well cared-for. An experienced oncology nurse once described this facet of the clinical encounter as the *fragrance of care.* It is not reliant on what you are doing with the patient or saying to the patient, but rather speaks to an ineffable presence that conveys that they have arrived in a safe space, wherein caring, compassion, and concern are steadfast and unyielding.

Therapeutic Humility

This domain speaks to those themes wherein *therapeutic approaches* and *personal growth and self-care* are indivisible; that is, elements of both domains are intrinsic to the nature of these particular themes. In essence, these themes speak to instances when the therapeutic approach is essentially defined as an opportunity to bring forward some specific personal qualities into the clinical encounter as a means of achieving optimal therapeutic efficacy. This hybrid domain is comprised of nine themes, including:

- Tolerating clinical ambiguity
- Trusting in the process
- Avoiding the urge to fix
- Sitting with the patient's emotional distress
- Accepting and honoring client as expert
- Being a catalyst for therapeutic change
- Modeling healthy processing of emotion
- Not avoiding emotion
- Being able to explore difficult topics

These themes speak to clinicians being able to endure and cope with significant emotional intensity while tolerating clinical ambiguity and uncertainty and relinquishing the idea that that they are necessarily there to fix or resolve issues. This domain, collectively labeled *therapeutic humility*, acknowledges that there are problems and challenges that defy solutions or, by their nature, are simply not resolvable. The texture of therapeutic humility is defined by a willingness to enter into difficult or ambiguous clinical encounters while relinquishing the idea that one brings easy solutions or answers. Therapuetic humility demands that the clinician be comfortable taking a nondirectional, nonauthoritarian stance. This domain underscores the need for the clinician to be humble and nonpretentious, to acknowledge the patient's expertise, and to trust in the therapeutic process.

In reflecting on the idea of honoring the client as expert, Dr. Woelk told the story of his father, who died when he was 82 of a glioblastoma, a brain cancer.

To put things into context, my dad was born in Russia and came to Canada out of the Ukraine in the 1950s. He came with nothing but a small suitcase of items and a $500 travel debt, which back then that would have been a lot of money. He didn't have much education, but he worked hard to look after his family and, like all of us wanted his kids to be successful. About 7 or 8 years before he died, he developed a bladder condition that ended up requiring the removal of his bladder and the creation of a urostomy. Considering the idea of dignity, losing that ability and requiring a bag was very difficult for him. I remember him telling me that he once complained to his doctor that the bag had fallen off in a restaurant and that it had been extremely embarrassing. The doctor's advice was to make sure he was always carrying an extra set of clothes. My dad didn't think that that was very helpful at all.

He did get really good care from the ostomy nurses, who offered him a number of different product options, and eventually found one that he managed really well. But then he was admited to hospital because he had been diagnosed with glioblastoma multiforma. He needed to be an inpatient because he had weeks of radiation and wasn't really able to function very well at the time. Early on in his stay his urostomy bag came off, so his nurse came to change the bag for him. He told her, "I do it this way." And she said, "No, I know how to do this. I've done this lots of times." So she did it. Then about 4 or 5 hours later, the bag came off and so the next nurse came on and she said, "I'll take care of this for you." And my Dad said, "When you do this, I noticed you're using a particular product to wipe the skin around the opening. You should use alcohol instead." She said, "No, here, we don't use alcohol, we use this product." And he said, "Well, at home, I always use alcohol," to which she replied, "well, here we don't. Here we use this product." So he was quiet. And again, about 4 hours later, the bag let go from the skin and she said she'd return to change it again. She seemed upset and unhappy with the situation, and my dad felt like she took it out on him, and then she repeated the process again. And, of course, when I arrived a few hours later, his gown was wet again and the room smelled some like urine.

I could imagine that my Dad would have been mortified about this. He was quiet and looking a little despondent, and he said that he was waiting, once again, for someone who would come again and address the leak. But there was a shift change, and he was still waiting. So this was a lack of dignity. The next person that came on was a nurse who said to my Dad, "well, I guess we're going to have to do this again." Now this nurse was fresh and at the beginning of his shift. And my Dad said, "You know, I do it differently at home." And he asked, "What do you do at home?" So my dad told him, "I use alcohol." "Okay," he says, "I'll go get some alcohol." So they put the bag on and, of course, 3 days later, the bag was still on. The next time I came in, he said, "You know what happened? One of the nurses came back, and she brought a whole bunch of young nurses with her and she said, 'this guy knows how to change his bag, and he does a really good job. So this time, we're going to let him do it, and we're all going to learn from him how it's done.'" For the remainder of his hospital stay, he was proud of his bag change day. Twice a week, a different group of young nurses would come in, and he would show them how to do it.

In reflecting on therapeutic humility, Dr. Harlos asks how one ought to behave "if you're blindfolded and parachuted into the middle of a crowded market square in some part of the world that you know nothing about. What would the wise person do? The wise person would be humble, observant, respectful, naïve, and curious. So anytime you walk into a room, that is what needs to happen in a matter of seconds. You are trying to get a feel for the culture of that room, a culture you know nothing about, and of those people. Some families, when you walk in there, have candles on the side, there's a bottle of wine, there's a big poster of this dad when he grew up and people are singing songs that were his favorites or they are praying at the bedside, or there is someone on the bed beside him. This is a celebratory room. Then there are the angry rooms. You walk in and no one looks at you, and everyone's got their arms crossed. You might notice in the culture of that family that there are front row, bedside seats, and there are the 'bleachers'—people at the edges of the room. So there is a sort of hierarchy. Are the bedside rails up or down, and are they holding hands or not holding the patient's hand? And all of this can be seen after you've only spent 5 or 10 seconds walking into the room, even before you've introduced yourself."

Therapeutic humility also acknowledges when the illness has the upper hand. For example, in his work as a pediatric palliative care consultant, Dr. Harlos encounters parents who are trying to make seemingly life-and-death decisions on behalf of their young children. "With adult patients, family can usually imagine what their healthcare choices might be when they can no longer communicate them based on their knowledge of their loved one. It's hard to say what a very young child would think, say because he is only 6 months old. But what I try to do is to say, 'You're being asked to make a lot of decisions, and it must feel like these decisions are about life and death, like deciding whether your child lives or dies. When we ask you 'Do you want to tube feed?' or 'Do you want this pneumonia treated or not?' or 'Do you want him on a ventilator or not?', those must seem like life and death decisions—if you decide not to have something done, it can feel as though you're choosing for your child to die. But I need you to take a step back and remember and reconnect with the fact that this illness, as we've said before, cannot be survived. There is no decision that we can put in front of you that will determine whether or not your child survives. We know that his life is on a path toward dying, and we're just asking you to help us choose the most comfortable path.'" Therapeutic humility acknowledges that there are things beyond the realm of our control.

In looking after women with gynecological cancers, Dr. Robert Lotocki often asks himself, "what if this was my wife, if this was my mother, if this was my daughter, how would I treat you? Most of the time, for many cancers you are using an algorithm of management that is somewhat mechanical. But you are trying to maintain a personal touch without making them feel that this is sort of a cookbook management. Sometimes you come back at the end of the day and see the patients, once everyone else is gone, and talk to them personally." In reflecting back on these conversations, Dr. Lotocki recalled the following case.

The patient was a 22- or 23-year-old young woman who had complications related to her cancer. She had a really nice personality, a nice family, but unfortunately she had a fistula, so stool was coming through her vagina so we ended up doing a palliative colostomy. That was something that she could accept and she kept hoping that, with ongoing therapy, the cancer would respond well enough that maybe we could reverse it. But her cancer just wasn't responding to treatment. As time went by she realized that her cancer was progressing and that she wasn't going to survive this. But to get there, she needed multiple conversations, which meant coming back to the bedside on multiple occasions. Many times you would say nothing. Those could be the longest silences in the world, but you are listening. You know she wants to say something that is bothering her, whatever it may be, so you listen. You don't have an answer at the end of the day but you listen. This helps her reach that final stage. She knows there is nothing that you can do. But dealing with that finality, meaning knowing she is not going to have the ability to survive, she is not going to have the ability to have kids, she is not going to have the ability to see her nephews and nieces grow up, and her parents are going to see their daughter die when the rule of thumb is that they should die before their kids. You help them deal with that, but mostly it is just listening because there are no answers. You don't have an answer as to why the cancer came in the first place. You don't have an answer as to why our treatments don't work for her particular cancer. We can put a person on the moon, we can put a person in space, but yet we can't come up with a treatment that is going to look after and treat her particular cancer.

This is the quintessence of therapeutic humility. It is marked by a willingness to be present in spite of not having a fix for the underlying health condition and being able to endure the emotional intensity of the clinical encounter. As Tom Roche points out, "to just be with someone's distress is incredibly difficult, partly because you need to be present with your own distress in order to be able to do that." You also need to trust the process, be able to sit with the patient's emotions, tolerate the ambiguity of the clinical enounter, and know that there are no clear answers.

Denise Klassen describes a similar situation, illustrating the importance of therapeutic humility, wherein showing up is the de facto clinical task. "The patient was an older gentleman dying on the ward. They were a Jewish family, and there was a lot of family members in room. He was already comatose. You don't have much to say to the family. What are you going to tell them? But you simply need to be there with them, not fussing, not trying to smooth his pillow, but just be there, be able to sense their agony and wait with them while you can. That means a lot to them."

Being able to tolerate uncertainty is part of therapeutic humility. Dr. Bruce Martin reflects on "being afraid to ask the question of 'What do you fear most?' for fear you might not be able to deal with the answer. 'I fear that if I die tomorrow, my 10-year-old daughter will grow up without a father. She'll get pregnant when she's young and choose a bad partner, and I won't be there to help her.' So tell a young clinician there are going to be times when it is difficult to hear some answers but you need to know that we have all been uncomfortable in hearing responses. We have all been uncomfortable with things we have had to deal with or treat, and it's okay to be uncomfortable. It's okay to be uncertain, but you need to be comfortable with uncertainty and you need to be comfortable feeling queasy. The unfortunate thing is we teach our students what to do if the blood sugar is too high and that you have to be definitive if the creatinine leans over 500. And you better do something if the sodium is too low or the pregnancy test is positive and they are only 6 weeks and having abdominal pain. You have to know what to do. So we teach certainty, but we have to teach uncertainty and how to recognize emotional or clinical discomfort and how to be with that."

Death and grief are instances when the only thing one brings into the therapeutic encounter is *self*. Again this invokes the essence of therapeutic humility. There is nothing you can say to fix what has happened, but, by virtue of showing up and trusting in the process, you can provide comfort and compassion. Dr. Gingerich described a mentor, Dr. Cripe, who had an impressive ability to connect with patients. "It wasn't that he spent a lot more time with patients, but there was always just a little bit when you got the sense he was connecting with them on a different level than *just the doctor*. I remember one instance where we had actually just walked into a room where a patient had just died, and the family was all sitting around, and he walked into the room and just kind of stood there with a certain look in his eyes as he made eye contact with the family members, but also mainly stared at the patient, even though the patient had just died. I don't know how to quantify the look, but he had this look and it was a moment, a prolonged pause where he didn't say anything but he just sat there, as if he was taking in the essence of the person. And then there was a little bit of a sigh. You could just get a sense that it meant something to him, to be there, even though the patient was gone, but just to be there with the family and the patient for a little while. It wasn't very long, and I took away from it that being there, sharing that moment, can be exquisitely important."

Therapeutic humility is not only about what you do with a patient, but sometimes what you don't do. When she was working as a family doctor in Canada's far north, Dr. Orr recalled delivering a baby of around 26 weeks gestation in a remote village in the middle of the night.

The very premature baby was born alive, the mother was very young and the grandmother was sitting with her. I realized that we were many, many hours, a half day or a full day away from a center that could look after a 26-weeker, and that even if the baby had been delivered in a neonatal unit, and this was in the early '80s, the baby would not have survived, but of course in hospital there would be an attempt at resuscitation. So it was difficult because the baby was alive, and my instinct as a physician was to insert an umbilical catheter and attempt a resuscitation and call for an airplane: in other words, go through all the motions I was trained to do. But my gut told me that this was embarking on a process that would not only have no benefit but would be harmful because it would deny the mother and the grandmother the chance to spend some loving moments with this child that was going to die. So I basically bundled up the baby to put in the arms of the grandmother and sat with them for about 45 minutes until the child died. This is not the kind of care that is often talked about in medical school. We can't just be thinking about catheters and intubation, bags and airlines coming with neonatal resuscitation teams. Patients and families want care that attends to their needs for love, for generosity, for humanity, and the way we interact with people, in this case the mother, child and grandmother."

Therapuetic humility also acknowledges when you have made a mistake or were in the wrong. Dr. Woelk recalls "missing a case of metastatic breast cancer and the patient dying, and going to the patient's home to talk with her husband and her husband's family, who asked me for a family meeting. And we went through things, and I realized that it could have happened to anybody. I was a young doctor, but I went in there, humbly saying, 'I'm sorry that this has happened and I wish it would have gone differently.' I know I've rescued a lot of relationships that way, by being humble. I think that's an important thing to do, to be humble and to be able to say, 'I think I might be partly responsible for this. Or I'm part of the big machine that's partly responsible for this, and let's see how we can make this better.' I think that's part of dignity."

Achieving Optimal Therapeutic Effectiveness

The surface and deep dissection of this body of communication knowledge yielded the model of optimal therapeutic effectiveness (see Figure 3.2). This model provides insight into how we can achieve optimal communication with patients that achieves dignity in care. There is a task, there is a setting within which that task occurs, and there is *self*—the person we bring into the clinical encounter—which need to be considered. As in any anatomical dissection, understanding form informs function. As such, the model can be used to deconstruct clinical communication as well as provide a way to think about how to achieve optimal therapeutic effectiveness. Let us consider a number of case examples to see how this works.

Dr. Lotocki recalled a young 16-year-old patient with advanced ovarian cancer. "She was the same age as my baby son at the time. She was in the Women's Hospital, which wasn't air conditioned and this young kid was unfortunately not responding to chemotherapy. She had a nice family. Her mother had breast cancer, her dad was healthy, she had a super brother who was a little bit older than she was, in his early 20s. I was on call that weekend and somebody—somebody being me—had to come in and talk to the family about palliative care and no resuscitation because she wasn't responding to treatment." The therapeutic task was clear, albeit not an easy one: discuss goals of care and resuscitation status. The domain of *personal growth and self-care* is invoked by virtue of the fact that Dr. Lotocki recognized that this child was the same age as his own son, thus putting him in touch with his own fears, vulnerability, and helplessness. It is noteworthy that he received the call to come in for this conversation. Often such tasks are relegated to junior staff or the medical student on call. Clearly this was not his practice, and while someone else could have obtained a do-not-resuscitate order, Dr. Lotocki recognized that he played an important role in this tragic, unfolding human drama. "Well, I drove in that Saturday morning, and it was much like today, beautiful, sunny, and hot, to have a conversation that I didn't want to have but knew I needed to have. I asked the family to come down, and they were there by the time I drove in."

The stage for an excruciating conversation was thus set, with the right setting and the right people involved, each taking their places. There is another facet of this clinical encounter worth placing within the context of the model. One cannot entirely predict how these difficult conversations will go. Will the patient or their family become inconsolably distraught? Will someone try to hijack the agenda? Will anger, pain, and confusion derail the process entirely? Will everyone understand the information being provided, allowing for decision-making that will lead to the best quality-of-life outcomes? Despite these unknowns, in order to enter into such a clinical encounter, one needs to give up the idea of having total control of the outcome. This speaks to almost every theme subsumed within the domain of *therapeutic humility*, including *tolerating clinical ambiguity, trusing in the process, avoiding the urge to fix, sitting with the patients emotional distress and not avoiding emotion*, and *being able to explore difficult topics, accepting and honoring the patient as expert, recognizing that we can be a catalyst for change*, and *modeling healthy processing of emotion*. In otherwords, Dr. Lotocki needed to accept, by way of walking into that room that beautiful summer afternoon, that he was not entirely in control, nor could he necessarily predict the outcome of this pending clinical encounter. "It actually turned out to be one of the easiest conversations that I have had about palliative care because she actually took over. I basically started painting the picture that this cancer is progressing and our therapies are exhausted and our next step was palliative care. I could see her parents turn white because they knew with the words being said that she was going to die and that resuscitation would not help her. But she took over the conversation by giving the example of a kid at school who fell off the back of a pickup truck, had a head injury, and was put on and virtually died on the respirator. She was able to use that analogy with her parents while I was in the room to say 'you don't want that for your daughter.' So it turned out to be easier than what I anticipated, because a 16-year-old girl took over." This is what optimal therapeutic efficacy looks like. Know the task, be mindful of the pace and what people are prepared to hear; set the stage to optimize safety for everyone; and, critically, being sure that you show up by way of bringing elements of who you are into the clinical encounter.

Dr. Gingerich recalled an example which is in stark contract to Dr. Lotocki's approach to determining resuscitation status. "I was a first-year resident in internal medicine, and we were on the wards late at night. A patient had just been admitted with some kind of serious illness, and it was our job to talk with him about his code status. I had just started, and there was a resident with me and he was showing me how to do it." So the therapeutic task was clear: determine code status. There were some red flags, however, given that this delicate conversation was about to take place in the absence of any kind of prior therapeutic relationship. "We walked into the room, and he was standing up looking down at the patient." Again there are red flags. Standing over the patient accentuates the power differential and conveys the message, "I don't really have time to talk with you," which can easily be interpreted to mean "you are not worthy of my time."

"He just jumped in with, without any sort of small chat or relationship building: 'well, if your heart or lungs stop, what would you like done?' And before the patient could really even answer that question, he jumped in to say, 'Well, I don't think it would be very helpful to do this, I don't think we should do this,' and within a few seconds the whole conversation was done and he walked out. It felt like coercion, like he was pushing the patient into making a decision, without a whole lot of back and forth. There wasn't much dignity in this throughout."

Although strictly speaking the therapeutic task was accomplished and the code status was obtained, the opportunity for optimal therapeutic efficacy failed miserably. No attention was paid to establishing a safe milieu, no attempt was made to establish any kind of relationship or connection, and no element of *self* was brought to the bedside. There was a complete lack of awareness of the pathos and emotional resonance that asking someone to forgo life-sustaining treatment entails. Even small nuances would have made a difference. Sitting instead of standing, asking how they are doing this evening, acknowledging that "this must be so difficult." Dr. Gingerich believes that "the medical conversation needs to include letting the patient know that *I am there with them through this process*, even just showing a facial expression, a small empathic statement that lets them know that I recognize their suffering." If we regard patients strictly as the embodiment of their illness, code status becomes a technical task. If, on the other hand, we recall that *patients are people with feelings that matter*, determining if someone will provide consent to forgo measures that are meant to prolong life requires a thoughtful conversation and deserves to be conveyed in a fashion that optimizes therapeutic efficacy.

Dr. Jeff Sisler recalled some instances when optimal therapeutic communication was woefully lacking. The first was the case of a woman in her mid-70s who struggled with feeling dismissed by her neurosurgeon. While he was seemingly technically competent, she reported feeling afraid and fearful of this surgeon. "He stood up in his white lab coat, didn't make eye contact, and dropped a coin on the table and said 'it's a 50/50 proposition' as to whether she would be paralyzed from the surgury as opposed to being helped by it. While she had the surgery, which went fine except for some remnant chronic pain, she and her husband were nevertheless terrorized by that." While the surgeon conveyed the fact that this operation was high risk, he did so in a way that emotionally assaulted the patient rather than making any attempt at establishing a therapeutic connection. While he cryptically conveyed prognostic information, there was no attention paid to patient safety nor any evidence of invoking therapeutic pacing, presence, or humility.

Dr. Sisler recalled another case that was referred to him after the patient switched providers because they were not happy with their previous physician. "The patient was an older woman, who was very earnest and tearful as she talked about her prior visit. The oncologist apparently opened the door and within a few seconds said 'the scans show the disease is terminal and you've got 6 months to live,' which sounds like a bad movie. The patient felt like she'd been slapped in the face, being appalled and frightened. I prescribed chemotherapy for her metastatic cancer, and she received one cycle and lived for close to a year, and it was decent, I think she would have said that it was a year worth living." Again, while the oncologist she saw first disclosed prognostic information, none of the other elements of optimal therapeutic efficacy was paid heed, resulting in a complete rupture of the clinical relationship.

Sue Bates recalled a clinical anecdote which epitomizes falling short of optimal therapeutic communication. The patient was a "woman with breast cancer who was scheduled for bilateral mastectomy and full reconstruction. Her physician then got back some results from a PET scan, indicating that she had metastatic disease. He just rang her up over the telephone and told her, 'You're not having surgery, it's all cancelled now. You can't have this because you're metastatic and you're going to die.' It happened, and there is no dignity there." While the designated task was the sharing of prognostic information, the way in which it was done illustrates striking therapeutic failing on every possible level. A telephone conversation can be less conducive to the creation of a safe space in which emotionally evocative information can be shared. There are no assurances who the patient is with, or who they have to support them as they receive this information. Telephone contact also leaves little room to establish or convey therapeutic presence: in the absence of personal contact, it is much more difficult, albeit not impossible, to convey respect, genuiness, authenticity, trustworthiness, and presence.

The abrupt and crass pronouncement of a change in therapeutic plans and prognostic outlook suggests that no attention was paid to the matter of therapeutic pacing, with nothing being done to gauge what the patient knew, what they wanted to know, and what they were ready to hear. Perhaps the single most egregious failure in this startling vignette was the absence of elements contained within the domain of personal growth and self-care. Anyone sharing this kind of difficult information must be mindful of the psychological and existential enormity of such a task, and how what you are about to say will change someone's life and that of their family and community forever. It behooves the messenger to be in touch with how this might feel and what this might mean to patients, which means reflecting on how they themselves or those they love might react in similar circumstances. Being mindful of this will not always guarantee that you will find the right words, but, more importantly, it will almost invariably ensure that you strike the right tone. And so, in a setting that offers you and the patient some privacy, you might find yourself saying something like "There is a difficult conversation we need to have. Is this a good time to talk? Your results are back, and I'm afraid the news isn't good. I wish I didn't have to be telling you this, but I'm afraid your cancer has spread. We need to plan together our next steps in dealing with your illness. I know I have covered a lot, and you may have questions, now or perhaps later, that you will want to ask me. When you've had a chance to absorb all of this, and talk it over with your family, let's arrange a time to speak again." This is not meant so much as a script, but rather as an emotional template, demonstrating that you care about this news, that you are not indifferent to how devastating this is, that you are sensitive to the amount of information that can be absorbed at any given time, that despite the change in outlook, you remain involved and committed in your role as a care provider.

Sue Bates speculates that sometimes healthcare providers, and especially physicians, overlook these elements of care and communication. "I think that they have forgotten. Some of them are so focused on doing a particular piece of research, or they've got this number of patients coming into clinic, or they've got teaching tomorrow. They have everything delivered to them. The notes are there, the chart is placed in front of them. They rarely even have to come out and bring the patient into the room. When all of this is done for them, it gets to feeling like a conveyor belt, and they forget the person sitting in front of them. I don't think some of them cope with the reaction of some patients, who may get angry, tearful, or very emotional, and so it's like they switch off, perhaps as a coping mechanism to get through it."

When the therapeutic task feels particularly ambigious, paying attention to pacing and invoking therapeutic humility become front and center. Dr. Jonathon Wong is a young and talented internist on the palliative care service with the Winnipeg Regional Health Authority. He describes himself as someone who thinks fast, talks fast, and is the epitome of clinical efficiency. One day, still early in his tenure as a member of the palliative care house staff, he was called to the emergency department to see a middle-aged woman with advanced metastatic breast cancer. Over the previous week she had stopped talking, and there was concern that the cancer might have spread to her brain. Given that ours is a teaching service, Dr. Wong asked a rotating resident and medical student to accompany him. He found the patient lying on a gurney, with several worried family members hovering by her side. After a brief examination, during which the patient remained mute, Dr. Wong decided to sit down at her bedside for a few minutes and "do a mind meld." He explained that this was an attempt to slow himself and the process down and try to imagine what she might be thinking or feeling. Having decided he would transfer her to the palliative care ward, he stood up, took her hand, and said, "we will take care of you." Much to his surprise, she briefly opened her eyes and, for the first time in days, spoke, with the response, "Thank you." Seen through the lens of the model of optimal therapuetic communication, his task was to determine if she was a candidate for admission to palliative care. Given that he was told she was mute, the communication agenda was entirely nebulous. By trying to imagine the patient's experience, Dr. Wong was bringing something of himself into the clinical encounter, contemplating what it might feel like to be frightened or confused or simply absent. He purposefully slowed down the pace, spending a few quiet moments at her bedside, acknowledging within himself that, despite his inclination for speed, this situation called for a different approach. As in previous examples, therapeutic humility saw him yield to the uncertainty of the process, tolerating its ambiguity and its far from certain outcome. The combination of these elements yielded a brief, albeit extraordinary outcome, for which he was miraculously thanked.

References

1. Chochinov HM, McClement S, Hack T, McKeen N, Rach A, Gagnon P, Sinclair S, Taylor-Brown J. Healthcare provider communication: An empirical model of therapeutic effectiveness. Cancer. 2013;119:1703–1713.
2. Palmer PJ. Introduction: Teaching from within. In: *The courage to teach: Exploring the inner landscape of a teacher's life*. Jossey-Bass; 2017:1–8.
3. Frazee C. "The vulnerable": Who are they? https://www.virtualhospice.ca/en_US/Main+Site+Navigation/Home/For+Professionals/For+Professionals/The+Exchange/Current/%e2%80%9cThe+Vulnerable%e2%80%9d_+Who+Are+They_.aspx

The Stone Angel

So, if this were indeed my Final Hour, these would be my words to you. I would not claim to pass on any secret of life, for there is none, or any wisdom except the passionate plea of caring. . . . Try to feel, in your heart's core, the reality of others. This is the most painful thing in the world, probably, and the most necessary. In times of personal adversity, know that you are not alone. Know that although in the eternal scheme of things you are small, you are also unique and irreplaceable, as are all of your fellow humans everywhere in the world. Know that your commitment is above all to life itself.

— Margaret Laurence

Laurence M. *The stone angel*. McClelland and Stewart; 1964.

4
Dignity in Care

Previous chapters covered what shapes patients' responses to changing health circumstances and the importance of dispositional attributes described in the ABCDs of dignity-conserving care. We have also examined an empirical model of therapeutic effectiveness that allows for optimal connectedness and sensitivity in communicating with patients and their families. But to understand and achieve dignity in care, we need to be mindful of the multitude of factors that can bolster or infringe upon patients' sense of dignity.

Most healthcare providers and their professional associations would espouse to offer care that is mindful of and responsive to patient dignity. The Canadian Medical Association Code of Ethics and Professionalism proclaims, *always treat the patient with dignity and respect the equal and intrinsic worth of all persons.* It's American counterpart, the American Medical Association Principles of Medical Ethics states that, a *physician shall be dedicated to providing competent medical care, with compassion and respect for human dignity and rights.* In a very similarly worded statement, the World Medical Association Code of Medical Ethics states that a *physician shall be dedicated to providing competent medical service in full professional and moral independence, with compassion and respect for human dignity.* The Canadian Nurses Association Code of Ethics says that *it is important for all nurses to work toward adhering to the values in the Code at all times for persons receiving care—regardless of attributes such as age, race, gender, gender identity, gender expression, sexual orientation, disability, and others—in order to uphold the dignity of all.* The Canadian Association of Social Workers Scope of Practice Statement says, *principles of respect for the inherent dignity and worth of persons, the pursuit of social justice, and culturally responsive practice that applies an anti-oppressive lens to all areas of practice and is grounded in ethics, values, and humility, are central to social work.* In June 1964, the World Medical Association issued the Declaration of Helsinki, which states, *It is the duty of physicians who participate in medical research to protect the life, health, dignity, integrity, right to self-determination, privacy, and confidentiality of personal information of research subjects.*

Despite the apparent centrality of dignity in these lofty policy statements and codes of ethics, there is very little guidance on how to instill dignity into day-to-day clinical practice. Dr. Orr suggests that the essence of dignity in healthcare resides in "recognizing the uniqueness of the individual, resulting in them feeling that they are seen, accepted, and embraced for who they are. This means having to strip away my own biases and, to some extent, my own values, using all of my senses and full capacity to see, hear, and feel the humanity of that person." Dr. Bruce Martin describes dignity as "the foundation of how I provide care. This isn't unique to palliative care, but speaks to the relationship between myself as a healthcare provider and an individual and their illness, meaning the experience they are having, the journey they are taking with their illness, and the impact it is having on their life and their family. I try to weave this approach to care based on what I have learned and understand of their life and their family, and how they fit within their broader community. It's as simple as *caring*. As institutions we are quite capable of providing the medical knowledge and foundation to provide care. We are less good at modeling caring. So we need to make sure that we care about, and not just provide care for, our patients."

The Case for Dignity

Why are considerations of dignity so important and worthy of our collective attention? Perhaps the most convincing evidence comes from empirical studies that have examined the association between perceptions of dignity and a wish to die. These studies affirm that loss of dignity is a strong predictor of desire for death and one of the most highly cited reasons why patients seek out euthanasia or assisted suicide. One study reported that, according to Dutch physicians who had complied with their patient's wish for a hastened death, loss of dignity was the most frequent reason driving their request.[1] It would thus appear that there is a profound existential connection between dignity and a wish to go on living, and, in its absence, patients may feel life is no longer worthwhile. Little wonder that in our studies of dignity in patients nearing death, those with a fractured sense of dignity were significantly more likely to report a strong desire for death and loss of will to live, along with depression, anxiety, and hopelessness.[2] Loss of dignity would appear to be a final common pathway wherein fractured dignity undermines will to live and bolsters a wish to die, sometimes leading to a decision to hasten death. While these studies tell us that dignity is profoundly important, even foundational to sustain a wish to carry on living, what they don't tell us is how to support, maintain, or even bolster dignity for those who find it under assault.

The Model of Dignity

So how do we put dignity into practice? Definitions such as this slight adaptation put forward by the World Federation of Mental Health captures the essence of dignity:

> Dignity is the inherent and inalienable worth of all human beings, irrespective of age, social status, race, ethnicity, religion, gender, sexual orientation, physical or mental state.

This wonderful definition, however, does not describe how we can direct our practice to the preservation of patient dignity. Hence, we turn to the empirical Model of Dignity in the Terminally Ill, which resulted from a program of research aimed at explicating dignity within the context of life-theatening and -limiting conditions.[3] A cohort of 50 dying patients was interviewed, asking them detailed questions about how they understood the term "dignity" within their particular circumstances, what experiences supported or undermined it, and how it was connected to their sense of life being worth living.

While this model was based on detailed interviews with dying patients, their perspectives may have applications for anyone grappling with significant life-altering or life-limiting medical conditions. In essence, the model indicates that there are three broad domains that one must be mindful of and attentive to in order to achieve dignity in care. These include Illness-Related Factors, the Dignity-Conserving Repertoire, and the Social Dignity Inventory (see Figure 4.1).

The Patient Dignity Inventory

Based on the Model of Dignity in the Terminally Ill, we developed a 25-item distress screening instrument coined the Patient Dignity Inventory (PDI) (see Box 4.1).[4] Unlike many other screening instruments, the PDI is multifaceted and taps into physical, psychosocial, and existential/spiritual domains of patients' experiences that may influence their sense of dignity. The PDI invites patients to rate the degree to which they find various issues

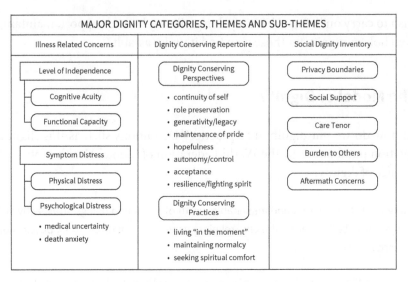

Figure 4.1 Model of dignity in the terminally ill.[3]

problematic, ranging from whether they are having distessing symptoms or feeling depressed or anxious, feeling a burden to others, or simply no longer feeling like they are the person they once were. The PDI has been translated into more than a dozen languages and can be used to tap into what patients are experiencing, provide them language to express those experiences, and even track those experiences over time. In a study reporting on 429 PDI responses from patients with cancer, healthcare providers indicated that in 76% of instances it revealed something about the patient they did not previously know. In addition to its utility in identifying dignity-related distress, the PDI enabled clinicians to provide more targeted therapeutic responses to areas of patient concern.[5]

Unpacking the Model of Dignity

Illness-related concerns refer to those influences that derive from and are directly related to the illness itself and that threaten to impinge on the patient's sense of dignity. The defining characteristic of these issues is that they are illness-mediated and directly related to the patient's illness or healthcare experience. This model category subsumes two themes, including Level of Independence and Symptom Distress. The first, Level of Independence, includes Cognitive Acuity and Functional Capacity. These implicate the

Box 4.1 The patient dignity inventory.

Patient Dignity Inventory

For each item, please indicate how much of a problem or concern these have been for you within the last few days.

1 = NOT A PROBLEM   3 = A PROBLEM   5 = AN OVERWHELMING PROBLEM

2 = A SLIGHT PROBLEM   4 = A MAJOR PROBLEM

1 Not being able to carry out tasks associated with daily living (e.g. washing, getting dressed).

2 Not being able to attend to my bodily functions independently (e.g. needing assistance with toileting-related activities.

3 Experiencing physically distressing symptoms (e.g. pain, shortness of breath, nausea).

4 Feeling that how I look to others has changed significantly.

5 Feeling depressed.

6 Feeling anxious.

7 Feeling uncertain about my health and health care.

8 Worrying about my future.

9 Not being able to think clearly.

10 Not being able to continue with my usual routines.

11 Feeling like I am no longer who I was.

12 Not feeling worthwhile or valued.

13 Not being able to carry out important roles (e.g. spouse, parent).

14 Feeling that life no longer has meaning or purpose.

15 Feeling that I have not made a meaningful and/or lasting contribution in my life.

16 Feeling that I have "unfinished business". (e.g. things that I have yet to say or do, or that feel incomplete).

17 Concern that my spiritual life is not meaningful.

18 Feeling that I am a burden to others.

19 Feeling that I don't have control over my life.

20 Feeling that my health and care needs have reduced my privacy.

21 Not feeling supported by my community of friends and family.

22 Not feeling supported by my health care providers.

23 Feeling like I am no longer able to mentally cope with the challenges to my health.

24 Not being able to accept the way things are.

25 Not being treated with respect or understanding by others.

Chochinov et al JPSM 2008

patient's ability to think rationally and coherently and to carry out usual routines, respectively. What we do and our ability to rationally navigate our way through those day-to-day routines can have profound implications on our sense of dignity. Loss of independence can lead to feelings of being a burden to others, undermining one's sense of dignity.

In a study of 253 palliative care patients using the PDI to examine the landscape of dignity-related distress, the inability to carry out normal routines was ranked most highly at 51.4% (see Table 4.1).[6]

Recall the young patient who left his wife during the course of his cancer treatment because he could not tolerate the idea that he would not be able to *be the man of the house*, which meant attending to household chores including *carrying in the groceries*. Clearly, the inability to carry out these seemingly banal tasks struck at the core of his sense of self and existential integrity. This same landscape study reported that 20% of patients experienced *not being able to think clearly* as a significant source of dignity-related disress (see Table 4.1). A 59-year-old woman with metastatic breast cancer described the effects of experiencing diminished cognitive capacity on her sense of dignity. "The 4 or 5 weeks I was on morphine . . . I'm not aware of that time in my life at all . . . lost it completely. I've seen pictures of myself at the table having Christmas dinner and I don't even remember Christmas. Who was here? And I have a feeling I might have said something to a couple of people and yet I can't bring myself to ask them if I did . . . so in that real case, I lost my dignity."[3]

Symptom distress refers to the discomfort or anguish that one can experience as a result of the underlying health condition. The landscape study found that 48% of patients reported that physically distressing symptoms were a significant source of dignity-related distress (see Table 4.1). The connection between symptom distress and dignity is that physical anguish can weaken resolve and truncate autonomy while threatening bodily and emotional integrity. Persistent or severe symptoms easily become an overwhelming preoccupation, undermining agency and a wish to go on living. In describing his perception of dignity, a 50-year-old man with advanced colon cancer and liver metastasis shared the following: "To die in peace . . . not suffering too much. Because toward the end, that's when people seem to suffer the worst. Just before the end. It's not emotional pain. It's real pain. Sometimes I hurt so much, I'd like to take all my pills and get it over with so I wouldn't hurt."[3]

While symptom management isn't typically thought of as a dignity-alleviating intervention, the data affirm that vigilance and attentiveness to symptom distress can alleviate or prevent a fracturing of dignity. I recall a

Table 4.1 Prevalence of distress in palliative care

PDI item	Percentage with problem
Not able to continue usual routines	51.4
Physical distressing symptoms	47.8
Not able to carry out important roles	37.5
Feeling no longer who I was	36.4
Not able to perform tasks of daily living	30.4
Feeling of not having control	29.2
Feeling uncertain	26.9
Not able to attend to bodily functions	26.5
Feeling anxious	24.5
Feeling of reduced privacy	24.5
Feeling a burden to others	24.1
Feeling how you look has changed	22.5
Feeling depressed	22.5
Worried about future	20.9
Not being able to think clearly	20.2
Feeling of unfinished business	19.4
Feeling life no longer has meaning or purpose	17.4
Not feeling worthwhile or valued	17.0
Feeling have not made meaningful contribution	11.9
Not feeling able to mentally fight illness	11.9
Not being able to accept things as they are	11.5
Concerns regarding spiritual life	6.3
Not being treated with respect	2.8
Not feeling supported by healthcare providers	2.0
Not feeling supported by friends or family	1.6

patient who asked me to kill her because the pain was more than she could bear. When her pain was brought under control, she wanted nothing more than to be discharged home so she could spend time with her family on their horse ranch.

The other dimension of symptom distress is *Psychological distress*, which subsumes medical uncertainty and death anxiety. *Medical uncertainty* refers to the distress of not knowing, or being unaware of various aspects of one's health status or treatment. Our research found that 27% of patients reported that uncertainty was a significant source of dignity-related distress (see Table 4.1). Not being able to anticipate what the future might bring can undermine a patient's sense of dignity and security. Uncertainty can make it difficult to predict what tomorrow might look like in terms of their unfolding clinical condition, leaving them prey to a fate beyond their control. This kind of uncertainty can heighten insecurity and feeling a victim of an illness run amok. Dr. West describes patients he was operating on "for acutely ruptured brain aneurysms. There is a considerable risk that no matter how the surgery goes, these patients are going to have some deficit from vasospasm, a reaction to the aneurysm rupturing that is going to occcur in 7 or 8 days. There is a difference between walking into their room on day 9, with the patient saying, 'Why didn't anybody tell us that this was going to happen? Who missed what or who didn't do what? Why didn't anyone warn us?' It is very different when you have told them that 'this is likely going to occur and we are aware of it. We are treating you to mitigate this, but despite all of this, it is likely going to happen.' And so you walk in on day 9 and you say, 'You have vasospasm,' and they say, 'Well, yes, you told us that this was going to happen.' It is a totally different picture. They need to be aware of what the possibilities are."

Dr. Harlos also addressed the issue of medical uncertainty in the context of palliative care. "Let's say you come into your wife's hospital room and she is no longer eating or drinking much in the last few days. Well, anyone would recognize that upsets families. I ask our trainees, what is the prevalence of not eating or drinking much as you progress toward dying? It's 100%. What's the prevalence of families being concerned about that? It's 100%. So if you know something is going to happen 100% of the time, and you know it's going to bother people 100% of the time, why wait for families to come to you, asking why she's not eating her tray? You should be having those conversations well ahead of time." Information and forwarning provide a way of being able to assuage medical uncertainty, providing patients and families with the ablity to anticipate—and hence prepare for—what lies ahead.

One of the most frequently downloaded articles on the Canadian Virtual Hospice (virtualhospice.ca), authored by Dr. Harlos, is titled "When Death Is Near." This article describes in detail the process of what dying looks like and what patients and families can expect, with topics such as *decreasing energy with illness* to *final physical changes people might anticipate*. The popularity of this article attests to the fact that uncertainty and not knowing can be significant sources of distress and that informing people about their healthcare condition, being sensitive to what they want and are prepared to hear, can help restore patients' sense of dignity. This overlaps with *Death Anxiety*, which describes the worry or fear that is specifically associated with the process of death and dying. Again, the ability to ease this form of anxiety with sensitive, reliable, and well-titrated information is part of an overall dignity-preserving strategy.

Dignity-Conserving Repertoire

This second major category that emerged within the Model of Dignity refers to personal attributes or ways of being that can have an influence on patients' sense of dignity. Broadly speaking these issues can be divided into two themes including Dignity-Conserving Perspectives and Dignity-Conserving Practices. *Dignity-conserving persectives* refer to ways of looking at one's situation and the psychological or emotional attributes that help promote a sense of dignity. This theme is comprised of eight subthemes including (1) continuity of self, (2) role preservation, (3) generativity, (4) maintenance of pride, (5) hopefulness, (6) autonomy/control, (7) acceptance, and (8) resilience/fighting spirit. *Continuity of self* refers to the sense that the essence of who one is remains intact despite the incumbrances of any healthcare challenge. This sub-theme affirms that, for dignity to persevere, *who we are* must prevail over *what ailment we have*. At its core, it is the idea that we are not defined by our illness. A 64-year-old woman with lung cancer and brain metastasis described this notion in terms of how she still viewed herself as someone worthy of respect. "To me a lot of it would be recognizing that you are still an individual, a person who has had a life. I guess it's being treated with respect. [That] would probably be a big thing, being allowed input and taking your requests seriously and your decisions seriously."[3]

Role preservation refers to the patient's ability to continue to function in, or value and identify with, roles that are or were perceived to be important and congruent with their prior view of themself. Jacques maintained the identify of a professional musician until his very dying day (see Chapter 1). About 1 year before his death, as part of his surgical treatment for oral cancer, skin and soft tissue had been taken from his forearm to rebuild his tongue. Being right-handed, this graft was taken from his left forearm. Sadly, albeit completely predictably, contractures set in causing him to lose the exquisite dexterity in his left hand and fingers, bringing to an abrupt end his ability to play music. Shortly before his death, I paid him a visit in his hospital room. I recall him being mildly confused but resting quietly and comfortably as he faced the final days of his metastatic cancer. At one point during our visit, a nurse entered his room, busily engaged in making notations in his bedside chart. "Did you know that Jacques was a professional violaist?" I asked her. I continued by saying, "He played with all the world's greatest classical soloists, including Heifetz, Horowitz, Rostopovich, and Ashkenazy," to name a few of the handful that I could recall off the top of my head. Two things then happened simultaneously. His nurse turned her attention to Jacques as she slowly put down his chart, and he broke out in a broad smile and, as I recall, full body blush, reveling in the indelible memory of those past breath-taking performances while basking in the affirmation of who he still was to his very core. While later doing my own charting, I overheard his nurse sharing what she'd learned about Jacques' glory days with her colleagues, and it struck me that, by changing her perception and broadening her appreciation for who this man really was, I had provided dignity in care.

Generativity/legacy borrows from the work of Erik Erikson, the German American developmental psychologist and psychoanalyst best known for his theory on the eight stages of psychosocial development of human beings. His seventh stage of psychosocial development is coined "generativity versus stagnation," with generativity denoting *a concern for establishing and guiding the next generation.* In developing the Model of Dignity in the Terminally Ill, patients sometimes indicated that dignity resides in the comfort of knowing that, after they die, they would leave behind something lasting and transcendent of death for those mourning their loss. This was often conveyed by way of highlighting the importance of their accomplishments, contributions, and connections to life, such as children or good work. For example, an 88-year-old woman with breast cancer and bone metastases responded to the question regarding what gave her life dignity in the following way: "The accomplishments of my children . . . I would love to see my grandchildren graduate. . . . I'm not in a hurry to go anywhere.[3]

Dr. Woelk described the importance of generativity in his care for a gentleman and his wife. "He and his wife were in their 70s. They had three grown kids, and he had a leukemia of some kind and he came into the hospital. He'd been in a few times with infections and other complications, but I realized that this one was more than the usual. His counts were lower than ever, and I didn't think he was going to pull through, and so I sat down with them and I said, 'You know, you have an opportunity here that many people don't. You're able to say things to your family that some people will never get a chance to say, and you need to take the chance to say them, if you want to say them.' I often use Ira Byock's example, to say those important things like 'I'm sorry, I forgive you, I love you. I'm going to miss you, goodbye.' When I came in a couple of days later, he had arranged to meet with his family and his grandchildren. He had blocked off a couple of hours at a time. And he met with them all individually and he told them what he saw as their strengths and their weaknesses, and his hopes for them. And the things that they might be able to do with their strengths and how to overcome their weaknesses. Can you imagine that? He did that with his three kids, and he had about four or five grandchildren, and he pulled them all aside and had a chance to sit with them all. It wasn't as sad as it was really meaningful. And sometimes humorous. At one point, he and the family were telling me about this, they said, 'We've all had our chances to say those important things, and Dad was still alert, and he was kind of joking a little bit. Then he said, oh, I forgot to say, there will be no PowerPoint at my funeral.' And his daughter looked at me with these big eyes, and she looked at her Dad, and she said, 'I've been working at that for the last 3 days.' It was really just kind of a thrill, you know, it was just a real conversation."

The notion of generativity is also the theoretical foundation of a novel individualized brief psychotherapy developed by our research team coined *Dignity Therapy*.[7] This form of existential psychotherapy was developed specifically for patients with life-threatening and life-limiting conditions. It enables people nearing the end of life to engage in a therapist-guided process tapping into issues that are particularly salient to their sense of dignity. For example: *What parts of your history are most important? What are the most important roles you have played and what did you accomplish? What are you most proud of? What still needs to be said to your loved one? What are your hopes and dreams for your loved ones? What have you learned about life that you would like to pass along to others? What advice or guidance would you want to share? Are there important words or instructions you would like to offer your family?* These questions provide a framework for a recorded conversation, which is transcribed and edited to create a tangible legacy document, recognizing that it will serve patients' generativity needs by way of transcending death itself.

To date, there have been nearly 100 papers in the scientific literature addressing Dignity Therapy, including various clinical trials, along with seven systematic reviews. The collective evidence indicates that, depending on the cohort and study design, Dignity Therapy enhances end-of-life experience and, for those who are particularly distressed, may assuage depression, anxiety, and desire for hastened death.[8] Even in the absence of overt distress, Dignity Therapy provides patients an opportunity to enhance their sense of meaning and purpose, creating a legacy document that will speak to their loved ones for generations to come.

Mrs. Ackerman was a beautiful, funny, proud Jewish mother and grandmother who completed her Dignity Therapy about 1 week before her death. Besides sharing her history, which included her upbringing in North End

Winnipeg and how she and her late husband first met, she shared the following wisdom in her legacy document:

> The best thing I have as a legacy to leave are my children and grandchildren. I don't care what anybody says. I am leaving three of the biggest treasures in the world, plus the accomplishments of their children. And good, good, good children. They are my treasures. I am so thankful to have gotten these darling, darling, wonderful people. When people mention my kids, they always comment on how nice and wonderful they are. You know how much that means? That means a lot to a parent. I've had a wonderful life. I was married for 54 beautiful years. I raised three amazing children and seven grandchildren. I've traveled the world. I was President of Hadassah Wizo. I'm an accomplished bridge player and am known for my baking. I want my kids and grandchildren to continue on the way that they are right now. I want them to be caring. I want them to keep having great loving feelings to one another. I believe that they do. Listen, they're kids. They're always caring about one another. I want them to care about others as well. What a wonderful life I've had. I've told my kids, nothing is 100%. You're never, ever going to be everything perfect. But let me tell you something, if I could wish all my loved ones what I have, it would be a perfect world. I wish them the kindness, love, and appreciation of one another. They have such goodness in them. I love you more and forever.

When she died her son wrote me the following email. "We want to thank you so much for the time and efforts you spend with our mom Lois. She passed away Saturday at home surrounded by her family. She was an amazing lady and we will treasure her story forever. Thank you from the bottom of our hearts for you taking the time to capture who our mom was! Sincerely, The Ackerman Family."

Hayden Dookeran was a vivacious, charismatic, and proud Trinidadian. At the age of 55, he completed his Dignity Therapy within a week of his death. Here is part of the document he left for his family.

> We were put on earth to reproduce and bring up our children in the best way possible. That is what we are supposed to do. There's no doubt about it for me. I mean they're the future of this earth. My daughters are my most important accomplishment. Nothing compares to having your own child, and I have two beautiful daughters and I'm thankful for that. Everything I've done has rotated around them, my whole life, everything is towards them. The last 6 years were tough but if you look at all my 56 years, there's a lot of good, definitely a good life. I have nothing to regret. I got this multiple sclerosis from nowhere, and it's just my time, that's all. I want my

daughters to know that no matter what's coming down the pipeline, I dealt with it because I knew I was accepting whatever happened. Whatever's going to happen, I accepted it and I dealt with it. I want them to know they can do the same thing with anything in life. Treat people like you expect to be treated and take care of your children. That's what life is all about. Do your best for your children and do your best for yourself, and your family will blossom. There's a lot of good people and very few bad people. They just have to find good people. I want my family to always be good people. You will survive and good things will happen.

As illustrated in these two documents, Dignity Therapy offers patients an opportunity to exercise their generativity needs by way of providing them a framework within which to share memories, express their love and affection, and convey hopes and wishes for people they care about most. Dignity Therapy can instill a sense of meaning and purpose, allowing patients to safeguard the well-being of those they will soon leave behind. This happens through the sharing of stories, expressions of heartfelt feelings, sometimes words of forgiveness or remorse, explanations for past decisions or even missteps, the imparting of wisdom, and occasionally guidance on how to live life without them. My patient, Adair Warren, is a 55-year-old woman with terminal multiple myeloma. She describes herself as a life-enthusiast, former teacher, swimmer, and cyclist who, in spite of everything, says she is currently happy, curious, and grateful. Upon completing Dignity Therapy, she wrote, "Dignity Therapy is now a part of the bridge from here to there, from living life fully to what remains at the end, a story. Thank you for helping me tell this story."

Maintenance of Pride

Maintaining pride refers to patients being able to sustain a sense of positive self-regard in the face of diminishing independence. The essence of this is self-respect, without which patients feel diminished in the eyes of others and in their own self-estimation. Dr. Martin recalls ways in which he tries to elicit clinical encounters that home in on those areas of a patient's life that were or remain a source of pride or personal identity.

When I look back I had a good mentor who took me on home visits as a medical student and taught me that the first 30 seconds as you come in the door are to look about meaningfully and use what you see to establish a relationship with the patient or with their family. So I use a few visual cues or triggers to start a conversation that might be distant from the disease but is closer to the person. For us, I think, understanding the disease part is easy. It's the illness and the illness experience of the individual and family that I like to focus on. So I look around to see if there are pictures of children and grandchildren and family clusters. I look at paintings, photographs. Was he or she in a military uniform? What kind of things are on the bedside table, and can I use those things as an introduction of myself to the patient by saying, "Do you enjoy poetry," if I see a book of poems on the bedside table. I remember a nursing student saying to me, "The first thing you said to him was what kind of aircraft did you pilot? How did you know he was a pilot?" "Well," I said, "there's a picture over there next to the coat cupboard with him standing next to an aircraft, with a hold on the pro-peller, and two photos of aircraft on his bedroom wall. It seems to me it would be a natural question to ask. If I ask him first what did he pilot, what did he fly, what was his favorite aircraft, it gets us on a level of understanding that is a lot more fun for him than scrolling through pain, nausea, vomiting, disorientation, and furthermore gives me an opportunity of him speaking to me, which lets me determine if he is oriented and knows what I am talking about." It also acknow-ledges things in the patient's life that he did and may continue to take pride in as part of his core sense of self.

Hopefulness

Hopefulness refers to the ability to see life as having a continued or sustained sense of meaning and purpose. For most of our lives, hope is coupled with future expectations, the hope that something will happen or that life will unfold in a particular way as time moves forward. Toward the end of life, hope begins to uncouple from future expectations and is much more about the here-now than what the distant future may hold in store. While patients who are ill may yearn for cure or restoration of their prior state of health or functioning, patients whose illness extends beyond the scope of cure em-brace hope of a different kind, one comprised of meaning and purpose or finding refuge from the exigencies of their underlying illness. When asked to describe hope, a 66-year-old woman with pancreatic cancer responded that it was about "looking forward to the main event of the wedding right now."[3] Cathy Bourne, a pediatric oncology nurse clinician, described the changing nature of hope as death approached. "Sometimes families come to realize that choosing comfort is not giving up. It is one of the hardest choices to allow someone to die with dignity, but hope comes in different forms. I had a discussion with a mom of a 4-year-old. While they intially had hoped for cure, they didn't get that. So now she hopes her child will be a vibrant little boy for as long as possible."

Being terminally ill does not mean relinquishing hope since, despite death's imminence, meaning and hope are often possible. In fact, among dying patients, hopelessness is most often endorsed by patients who are suffering from concurrent depression.[9] Dr. West recalled a patient, who was "a very vigorous young lady who had been fighting a malignant brain tumor for quite some time and had a recurrence."

> She visited the neurosurgeon, who talked with her about the fact that surgery for this recurrence may cause a visual field defect, and he described that defect. The patient was quite taken aback because there wasn't any such defect from prior surgery, so why would there be one now? The surgeon grew impatient with the fact that he was talking about a life-and-death surgery and she was worried about a visual field defect. She was asking "Will I be able to drive?" to which in a cut-and-dried way he responded, "probably not." Finally, he said something to the effect, "Why are you worried about a visual field defect? This tumor is going to kill you." She just walked out and said, "that is just incredible." She said, "I don't really need somebody to tell me that this tumor is going to kill me. I know that. I am looking for somebody to help me prolong my independent lifestyle." She actually refused to have surgery by that person. So I did the surgery, and she didn't end up with a visual field defect. I would emphasize that it is important that we acknowledge that patients understand what the outcome of a terminal cancer diagnosis is. They are not naïve about the fact that if they have lung cancer with metastases, they are not going to outrun this, they are not going to get cured. And they resent being reminded at every stage that they are dying. Offering hope means supporting them optimistically and giving them reasonable therapeutic opportunities and not feeling that you have to remind them, repeatedly, that this is just delaying the inevitable.

Autonomy/Control

Autonomy and control are distinct from functional capacity. The latter refers to a sub-theme contained within the broader domain of Level of Independence, which speaks to the degree of reliance an individual has on others. Autonomy and control, on the other hand, can be maintained even in the face of profound limited capacity in that these reflect the degree to which patients are able to exercise agency or have continued influence on their life or things that concern their life. Take, for instance, the case of an elderly woman who was the domineering, powerful matriarch of her family. Even on her death bed the mere wag of her finger had her family scurrying to meet her various sundry demands. Despite very limited functional capacity she was able to maintain agency and exercise choice—who was allowed to visit and when they were allowed to do so, including where everyone was allowed to sit around her bedside.

Dr. Bruce Martin recalls a case regarding hard choices and autonomous decisions. The story he told took place over 30 years ago, involving "a 40-year-old man, married and father of a couple of kids, living in a small remote and distinct cultural group of First Nations of about 1,400 people offshore in British Columbia."

> He made a conscious decision after chatting with me that he did not wish to leave his community for hemodialysis, knowing that his life would end, knowing that his children would lose him as a father. But he could not come to terms with having to leave the community for hemodialysis, and his peritoneal dialysis could no longer sustain his renal function for renal replacement. It was an intriguing journey for me to work with the patient, his family, and his community, the culture of the community with my fellow healthcare providers, including the local shaman, and the renal program that was in the urban centre some 1,500 kilometers away, over how to make a decision and how to deal with this fellow who had made a decision not to leave his cultural community.
>
> I often reflect back on it because it was a difficult decision for me as a relatively young physician, having only been out for a decade, of how to work through not only the decision-making, but work through it with the family, and them coming to decisions that would support his withdrawal from renal replacement; also helping all of them understand what this was going to look like in terms of symptoms and last few days, recognizing that I had very few clinicians who supported my decision. But I chose to take that journey. I didn't have to engage with his community, I didn't have to engage with the spritiual leaders of the community, I didn't have to engage with his children, but I chose to. I invested myself in more that just his symptom management. I could have chosen to manage his shortnesss of breath and his fluid overload one way or another, but I chose to treat him within the context of his community. And when I sat at his bedside, managing his dyspnea, I chose to talk about his life as a commercial fisherman.
>
> I had some people within the community who felt that I was assisting his death. He did die within about 10 days of the initial discussions, and what followed was a process called a *settlement feast*. Before an individual is buried there is

a settlement, meaning everybody gets together and talks about ill feelings in an open setting, and shares ill feelings so it can be settled and not continued before the deceased is buried, because there was ill feeling toward me by some individuals about his end of life journey. At the end of a settlement feast, individuals to whom there is ill feeling are given a gift. And so the family gave me a gift, a silver bracelet crafted in Bella Bella on Campbell Island, BC, engraved with a whale, eagle, and salmon. I was told that the Heiltsuk tribe used the three images to reflect their connection to the land, the sea, and their ancestors. I've worn it every day since as a reminder of my commitment to patients, to families, to communities. Now it has been suggested that if I didn't wear it, something horrible would befall me, but that was said in jest.

Dr. Harlos described another case in which an 87-year-old man excercised autonomy by deciding he wanted his ventilator discontinued and be allowed to die.

This was earlier in my palliative care career and it wasn't a common thing in palliative care. What was trickier was that he was completely awake and alert. He had multisystem failure from an amyloid disease, but was completely clear and on TPN, dialysis, cardiac pressor drugs, and ventilated and was saying enough's enough. I went down to talk with him and his family. He was awake and writing, and I said, "We can take you to the palliative care unit and give you some medications, you're going to be asleep and then we'll stop the ventilator and you will be comfortable and you will probably die within a few minutes." Then his daughter said that it's actually more complicated than that because he wants to die at home. I thought about it and said, "as long as we've got an IV, I don't see why we couldn't do this." I don't think that had ever been done in the city at home, so I checked with the region, with the College, and they had no qualms and said it seemed a reasonable thing to do. His daughter then said that it was even more complicated because he lives on a farm 2 hours out of town. He was born on the farm, his grandparents homesteaded the farm, he built the current building by hand, he dug the basement with a shovel and a wheelbarrow, and he wants to die in that room in the house he built.

So that was a bit trickier, but the next day we were in the back of an ambulance, taking the 2-hour drive out to the farmhouse to withdraw him. He was awake the whole time, he knew where he was throughout. I remember his son went into the fridge and got out this piece of watermelon, it actually looked kind of raunchy and even a bit moldy looking. He squeezed it into his dad's mouth and said, "See dad, I told you you'd get to eat this." Apparently the day his dad was admitted, the son had brought home groceries including this big watermelon. The dad was upset because it was too expensive, and "we can't afford that kind of luxury" and "I'm not going to get to eat that anyways." So he was mad that this money was spent and he was too sick to eat that kind of thing. So this was a symbolic gesture. I remember thinking, I'm not sure he died from the vent withdrawal or acute food poisoning from that watermelon."

What is clear is that this patient, with no functional capacity, was able to exercise his autonomy by taking control of his end-of-life choices, determining where and when he would die.

Acceptance

Acceptance refers to an internal process of coming to terms with or resigning to the reality of one's changing health circumstances. We conducted a study which asked 211 palliative care patients which of their symptoms or concerns they would ascribe to their sense of dignity (see Table 4.2).[10] Of these patients nearing end of life, 72% reported that *not being able to accept the way things are* was something they would affiliate with their sense of dignity. The challenge in accepting changes to one's health status is usually proportionate to the length or chronicity of the underlying condition and the extent to which it lays claim to function, capacity, and personhood. Minor and fleeting challenges are usual easier to accept and quickly accommodated. Not so the case when illlness becomes chronic or debilitating, especially when those capacities are central or foundational to personal identity. Studies looking at sudden changes in health status as a result of stroke, myocardial infarction, traumatic brain injury, or spinal cord compression report that suicidality is associated with a nearly seven times higher likelihood of depressive disorder, and, when treated, suicidality remits. When these suicidal patients were followed 3 to 24 months later, most were no longer suicidal. Acceptance, it would appear, is sometimes only slowly acquired over time.[11]

Our own studies have shown that patients with prognostic disavowal are most likely to experience underlying emotional distress, as demonstrated by higher rates of clinical depression.[12] Acceptance can become especially difficult for those who are nearing end of life. The story of Jacques reported earlier is a case in point. This middle-aged professional violaist with oral cancer struggled as much with the inability to play music as he did with the idea that he would die. While he gradually came to terms with the imminence of his approaching death, he continued to rail against the idea of living life

Table 4.2 Percentage of patients who ascribe various symtoms or experiences
to their sense of dignity

	Variable	Agree or strongly agree (%)
1	Not being treated with respect or understanding	87.1
2	Feeling a burden to others	87.1
3	Feeling you do not have control over your life	83.7
4	Not feeling you made a meaningful or lasting contribution	83.3
5	Not being able to independently manage bodily functions	82.9
6	Not feeling worthwhile or valued	81.4
7	Not feeling supported by your community	80.3
8	Not being able to carry out tasks of daily living	79.6
9	Not being able to carry out important roles	78.5
10	Not being able to think clearly	77.3
11	Feeling life no longer has meaning or purpose	75.1
12	Not being able to continue with usual routines	74.9
13	Not being able to mentally fight	74.5
14	No longer feeling like who you were	74.4
15	Not having a meaningful spiritual life	73.7
16	Not being able to accept things the way they are	71.6
17	Changes in physical appearance	66.4
18	Feeling your privacy has been reduced	65.9
19	Feeling depressed or anxious	59.7
20	Uncertainly regarding illness	59.2
21	Experiencing distressing symptoms	53.1
22	Thinking how life might end	41.7

in the absence of music. An 87-year-old woman with end-stage lung cancer said that "to die with dignity means they accept it. You kind of grow into this whole thing from year to year. You get wiser and you get to know what the consequences are and what you have to do."[3] Avery Wiseman introduced the concept of *middle knowledge*, which refers to patients being able to deny death in order to minimize the bleakness of their terminal prognosis while making plans for death by completing a will, arranging burial plots, and planning a funeral service. This concept of middle knowledge was important for several reasons: it suggested the benefits of denial in preventing us from being overwhelmed by death terror, thus allowing us to assimilate and even accommodate the reality of our deaths at a manageable pace, and it suggested that human nature and biology utilize denial in complex ways that are not uniformly detrimental to the process.[13]

Resilience/Fighting Spirit

Resilience or *fighting spirit* refers to the mental determination that some people exercise in order to overcome illness-related concerns, hence optimizing their quality of life. While for some patients acceptance is a dignity-preserving strategy, others rail against their illness in order to maintain their sense of dignity. A 73-year-old woman with metastatic breast cancer said that, for her, maintaining dignity meant not giving up. "Seems to me [some people] are giving up, not me. I wouldn't give up that easy. See I'm not the kind of person to give up that easy."[3] Resilience can express itself in multiple ways, whether doggedly seeking out life-sustaining therapies in the face of a tenuous prognosis or engaging in dignity-conserving strategies that do not let the illness become life-defining. The latter can be achieved in myriad ways that give our lives meaning and purpose, by engaging in opportunities that are life-affirming and emotionally and spiritually nurturing.

Like the rest of the Dignity Model, these dignity-conserving perspectives are nonhierachical and are expressed according to the unique characteristics of each and every patient and their illness experience. These qualities mediate or in some instances buffer the extent to which sense of dignity is influenced by the illness experience. They are in essence the psychological or emotional repertoire that people are endowed with, which can be invoked to stave off individual assaults to dignity and personhood. No perspective is necessarily more potent than another, and one or few of them may be as effective for one patient as engaging in many or all of them for another.

Dignity-Conserving Practices

Unlike the Dignity-Conserving Repertoire, which describes internal attributes that manifest as ways of experiencing the world, Dignity-Conserving Practices refer to personal approaches or techniques that speak to ways of being in this world. This consists of three sub-themes, including living in the moment, maintaining normalcy, and seeking spiritual comfort.

Living in the Moment

Living in the moment essentially involves focusing on immediate issues so as not to worry about or be overly preoccupied with the future. For many patients the future is full of uncertainties and unknowns. This can be anxiety-provoking, making *here-and-now* focused strategies an important way to assuage distress. A 76-year-old woman with metastatic breast cancer reflected on this by commenting that, "you can look out the window and see flowers growing or children on the street and hear somebody laughing . . . that makes life worth living. Right now the most important thing in life is to try to live every day and be considerably happy. And not try to let anything burden you down. Right, you know, try to enjoy the day as much as I can."[3] Another 67-year-old outpatient with breast cancer, reflecting on what gave her life dignity, shared this comment: "Just living from day to day. Enjoying time with my husband. And right now, you know, just enjoying this beautiful summer weather."[3] The essence of living in the moment aligns with mindfulness, which was first introduced into mainstream medicine by Jon Kabit-Zinn.[14] He wrote that "Ordinary thoughts course through our mind like a deafening waterfall." In order to feel more in control of our minds and our lives, to find the sense of balance that eludes us, we need to step out of this current, to pause, and, as Kabat-Zinn puts it, to "rest in stillness—to stop doing and focus on just being."[14]

This state of mindfulness can be critical for patients, allowing them to not incessantly worry about the future or ruminate about the past, but rather to live in the moment, as Buddhist scholar B. Alan Wallace says, *to practice stillness and calm.*[14]

Maintaining Normalcy

Maintaining normalcy refers to carrying out usual routines and maintaining usual schedules to the extent possible while coping with whatever challenges are being imposed by the illness experience. The ability to maintain normalcy is usually inversely proportionate to the severity of the illness or disease and its associated impairments. Although maintaining normalcy is closely related to living in the moment, there is a sense of continuous or routine behavior that helps patients in their day-to-day coping that charactierizes this sub-theme. A 69-year-old woman with metastatic lung cancer described her strategy for maintaining digity as follows: "Well, dignity means being able to get up and have breakfast with my grandchildren before they leave for school . . . and have supper with them. The simple things like having meals with them."[3] Another previous patient of mine had returned home after a long stint in hospital due to complications of advanced metastatic breast cancer. Having lived with pain and nausea that had disrupted the last few months of her life, she spoke about the everyday pleasure of her routine at home, which included waking up each morning, feeling the sun on her pale skin, and reading her newspaper on her backyard porch while savoring her first cup of freshly brewed coffee.

Seeking Spiritual Comfort

This sub-theme refers to the dignity-sustaining effect of turning toward or finding solace within one's religious or spiritual belief system. An 87-year-old woman with lung cancer described this as follows: "Dying with dignity means . . . that [you] will call to God. When you face death it's inborn in us that we have something else in us. We know that this life is not the end of it . . . and that is dignity . . . isn't that just wonderful that you have that feeling . . . the Holy Spirit . . . he guides us, and if I ever get into a little bit of fear you know, when I have this pain, that the faith never, never changes. I have never lost my dignity."[3]

Dr. Woelk recalls a patient he cared for "who was in her 80s, who developed lung cancer and had a lesion in her lung that was up against her heart. And so the chances were pretty high that it could invade into her heart and she could drop dead very quickly. She had other medical ailments and so she was pretty limited in terms of her mobility. I remember how calm and ready she was to die, and a lot of that had to do with her faith as to where she felt she was going. And the comfort of knowing that. Many of her friends had died already, and she was going to go meet them. And she had the support of the people around her, who were part of her faith community."

He remembered another patient "in his 20s with a brain tumour, married, no kids. I got a call back to the hospital and the nurses said, 'You need to come right away, this man has stopped breathing and we're bagging him.' He was a full code and wanted resuscitation. He refused to accept the fact that he was dying; he was sure that God was going to miraculously heal him. And so I came rushing down to the hospital and I walked into the resus room. Somehow about 15 family members had gotten in there, and they were all standing around him. Half of them were crying and half of them were praying. There were a few nurses in the room. I remember the nurse who was bagging him was crying. He was a young man, and we had cared for him for a while and it was very emotional for everybody involved. And at the height of that, one of the people there prayed that God would come now and heal this man. I stood in the corner and wanted to shrink away because I thought, 'Where is this going to go? Where's this going to end up?' And I was just quiet. I just thought, my role here is just to be quiet, because there was nothing I could do to intervene in this. And then, after a while, that same person said, 'You know, I think God has a different plan here.' At that point his family was ready to let go and we stopped bagging him. Of course, he was already gone."

For many patients, seeking spiritual comfort is not associated with religiousity, but rather is affiliated with a sense of meaning and purpose that connects them with something greater than themselves. According to an international consensus document, *Spirituality is the aspect of humanity that refers to the way individuals seek and express meaning and purpose and the way they experience their connectedness to the moment, to self, to others, to nature, and to the significant or sacred.*[15] For some, confronting death can also be a time of spiritual crisis. Dr. Woelk remembered "an elderly lady, around 80, who had been having symptoms since around November, and in December, had some tests and sure enough, it was clearly a metastatic pancreatic cancer. She saw the oncologist in January, who said, 'in your case, the best is palliative care, and we're not going to do anything, because it would be more harmful to you to have treatments.' So she went home and she tore everything past July off of her calendar, because he said 'your average survival is about 6 months from the time of diagnosis.' So she said, 'I'm just going to take everything after June off the calendar.' So she tore it off the calendar. She was a very devout Catholic lady, and I saw her in June and she was despondent. She was completely depressed. She thought God wasn't coming to get her. She wondered if she had done something terrible, and she couldn't figure it out. I asked her nurse to get her a new calendar with July and August on it and put some items on there, things which she could look forward to. I think we used a little bit of Ritalin and an antidepressant, and she lived another month or two and then died comfortably in the hospital. But that was, for her, a real spiritual crisis."

Like Dignity-Conserving Perspectives, Dignity-Conserving Practices can buffer patients from illness-related challenges or soul-crushing assaults on their sense of dignity. Those with more positive perspectives may be able to invoke more dignity-conserving practices, while those who are depleted or defeated by their illness may feel defenseless against the onslaught of their underlying illness or healthcare condition.

The Social Dignity Inventory

This major category within the model refers to themes that pertain to social concerns or relationship dynamics that enhance or detract from a patient's sense of dignity. In other words, while being ill can infringe on dignity in particular ways (Illness-Related Factors) and the experience can be shaped by intrinsic factors that are internally held (Dignity-Conserving Repertoire), there are influences external to the patient that can confer or withhold dignity, sometimes referred to as *attributed dignity*. According to bioethicist Daniel Sulmasey, attributed dignity describes the value that human beings confer on others by acts of attribution.[16] The following themes offer a framework for understanding these external or socially mediated forces that can shape human dignity.

Privacy Boundaries

Illness or even the most minor of healthcare concerns can result in infringements on patients' privacy. Loss of privacy is an early and ubiquitous hazard of becoming ill or needing medical attention. Examining or dealing with naked bodies, for example, may be routine within the practice of medicine, but for patients this is far from routine. Hence, healthcare providers must always be mindful that examination room doors are shut, curtains are drawn, and patients are draped appropriately. While privacy boundaries must sometimes be stretched, they must never be broken by attitudes that are insensitive, belittling, exploitative, or sexualized. Private conversations should also not be carried out in earshot of others who are not privy to what is being discussed.

Advanced illness or marked disability often results in the pushing of privacy boundaries, as illustrated by this 61-year-old woman with lung cancer, responding to what would take away her dignity: "Having that young woman come in here the other day was very, very hard on me. Or to ask her to do anything for me, I find it very hard to ask her anything, I don't know how to describe it. For one thing, I've never had too much self-esteem, I suppose, and I always preferred to meld into a wall. I felt more comfortable there . . . things like not being able to go to the washroom by myself. Oh to me, that would take everything away from me because I am so modest."[3] Loss of privacy often goes hand in hand with loss of independence, which requires others to lend their assistance. A 76-year-old woman with metastatic breast cancer lamented violations to her privacy, which she deemed a profound assault to her dignity. "Oh my God, maybe putting me on the toilet seat. These are private things, you know. I still feel like I like my privacy. Even for my sleeping in, it's kind of embarrassing if I'm still sleeping if they come downstairs. You know I've got to be up first and get dressed and be here."[3]

A study on adaptation to dependency with intimate hygiene for people with advanced disease reported that *participants' distress about receiving care with intimate hygiene was individually mediated, ranging from embarrassment at having another intrude into their personal space through to feeling humiliated, frightened, terrified, and wanting to die.*[17] Disability rights activist and scholar Dr. Heidi Janz reminds us that "there is nothing really inherently undignified about *needing* care; most often the loss of dignity that people associate with needing assistance with personal care actually stems from a lack

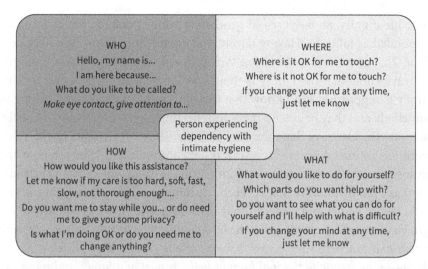

Figure 4.2 The who, where, what and how of providing assistance with intimate hygiene.[17]

of control over when, where, how, and by whom intimate care is provided" (personal communication, May 20, 2021)." To lack control means to loose agency, which is why people living with disabilities reliant on others for intimate care—bathing, dressing, toileting—emphasize the importance of facilitating autonomy by having their choices and preferences adhered to. This happens when carers *replace the participant's hands* and *assist with things the way the client needs it to be done.*[18] As patients move toward death, the need for intimate care is almost universal, given decreasing functional capacity. Even in these circumstances exquisite attention must be paid to dignity in care since patients experience helplessness when care is provided in a manner that thwarts agency (e.g., not asking patients who they want to assist them with intimate hygiene, how they want this handled, what they do or do not want assistance with) leading them to feel powerless and vulnerable (see Figure 4.2).

Opportunities to maintain control through active engagement and the ability to influence the receipt and provision of care is of critical importance in maintaining patient dignity.

Social Support

This sub-theme refers to the presence of an available and helpful community of friends, family, or healthcare providers. In responding to what gives your life dignity, an 80-year-old gentleman with metastatic prostate cancer responded as follows: "Having family. Having the little fellow that lives next door. That gives me a lot of cheer. Well it doesn't matter how bad things get. I always know that my family is there and I'm very lucky. Not everybody's family is supportive. But I know that they love me. Yeah, because I belong to somebody and they belong to me."[3] In reflecting on the importance of social support, Dr. Orr says that "the way patients define themselves in their humanity is intimately connected with others around them." She refers to the philosophy of *Ubuntu*, which is a Bantu term meaning *humanity* and is translated as *I am because we are*. A recent definition of *Ubuntu* describes it as *a collection of values and practices that Black people of Africa or of African origin view as making people authentic human beings. While the nuances of these values and practices vary across different ethnic groups, they all point to one thing—an authentic individual human being is part of a larger and more significant relational, communal, societal, environmental, and spiritual world.*[19] Dr. Orr explains, "this means we are only truly human in relationship to other people, and in the absence of other people, we are not fully human. So from this perspective, dignity means how one is seen and responded to by others around them." Having social support offers patients the opportunity to be with those who will provide help, encouragement, and, whenever possible, affirmation.

Dr. Woelk described an elderly lady he recently looked after and the importance of social support in sustaining her toward the end of her life. "She was about 90, and she had pancreatic cancer, and her kids came in. One of them from within the province, and two of them were from outside the province. They basically moved in to look after Mom, especially now with COVID and no visiting abilities at the hospital, so they were able to spend time with her. This family came thinking that Mom was going to die in the next month or two, and she ended up living around 3 or 4 months. They debated going to the hospital, but again, the visiting was going to be so limited, they decided to keep her at home and they did fine at home. This lady could not have done this at home without the support of her family. She died a very good death, surrounded by the ones she loved."

Care Tenor

Tenor refers to the tone of care, which speaks to those ineffable emotional and empathic qualities that infuse a clinical encounter and that are shaped by the health care provider. This implicates not so much what one does with or for patients and their families, but rather speaks to a way of *being* with them. Many facets of Care Tenor map onto the elements of therapeutic presence described in the Model of Optimal Therapeutic Effectiveness (see Chapter 3). That is, to set the tone of care, your way of being within the clinical encounter must emanate a *fragrance of care* that includes being compassionate and empathetic, being respectful and nonjudgmental, being genuine and authentic, being trustworthy, being fully present, being mindful of boundaries, being emotionally resilient, and valuing the intrinsic worth of the patient.

There are some practical and tangible things that can establish Care Tenor. To begin with, as Dr. West points out, "be on time and show respect for the patient's schedule. I see that a lot of patients come and wait for hours because they are willing to give up any amount of time to see the specialist or the family doctor, but that is not a very good management of everyone's time." It also conveys a message that *your (the patient's) time is not particularly valuable,* and *you being inconvenienced is none of my concern.* Dr. West also suggests that "the way you dress shows respect or not to the patient. You don't have to wear a tie, but I think you need to have a neat and approachable demeanor. I think that makes a difference to patients. I think it is part of the culture of respect because people have this expectation that nurses, physicians, people with responsibility are going to look as if they carry that responsibility. Those aren't the most important parts, but I think they can set the tone of the clinical encounter."

By way of example, Dr. West describes what a typical initial encounter might look like: "I will usually say, 'I am familiar with your case because I have looked at the records that were sent and I've looked at the x-rays, but I would like to learn a little bit about you. So tell me about yourself. For instance, what is your age and occupation?' I might ask a little bit about the family and holidays and things like that. It doesn't take much but it really lubricates the conversation. It's easy to talk about those things. People love to talk about themselves and their families. That doesn't take a long time, usually maybe 5 minutes out of a half-hour consultation. I think it shows the person that you are interested in them as a person, not just as a brain tumor or an aneurysm. It is so important that they also get to know what your intentions are and that you are going to do your best for them. This is especially true when you have the kind of situation like we have when somebody is impaired in terms of their cognitive function. There is a tendency to ignore them if you are talking to the daughter or the son. And the patient is there, and this is going on around them. Sometimes they are so impaired that you can't really include them in the conversation because they don't have the ability to answer the questions, but I always take time to learn just where they are and how comfortable they are with me talking to their family."

What Dr. West does not say, but is no doubt felt by his patients and their families, is that he has a way about him that makes the people he is with feel like they are the sole focus of his attention. He emanates an authentic, personal warmth and trustworthiness that makes you feel safe and cared for. In other words, his Care Tenor, his way of being with patients and families, his *fragrance of care*, embodies all of the elements of therapeutic presence (see Chapter 3), including compassion, empathy, and respect.

Burden to Others

The etymology of the word "burden" comes from the Middle English *burden, birden or burthen,* which means to *carry or bear a heavy load, responsibility or onus,* or *to cause worry that is grievous, wearisome or oppressive.* Patients who feel a burden to others are themselves burdened with the preoccupation that they constitute a heavy weight others must bear, that their very existence imposes unwanted responsibility or onus on others, and that they are the source of wearisome or oppressive concern for everyone within their circle of care. Feeling a burden is often associated with dependency and having to rely on others for various aspects of care. Given the association between autonomy, dignity, and personhood, it is little wonder that feeling a burden to others is often associated with feeling life is no longer of value and, depending on the intensity of those feelings, like life is no longer worth living. A 76-year-old patient with metastatic breast cancer lamented about the possiblity of being a burden to her children. "I wouldn't want them to take on the burden of doing that. That I have to depend on people just to look after me, to wash me, to take me to the bathroom and to cleanse . . . clean me up . . . I know this happens but I wish it didn't happen to me."

Our own studies of burden to others in terminal illness found that in a cohort of 211 patients, 23% reported severe ratings of burden to others, with the highest correlations being with depression, hopelessness, and general outlook. Further analysis of these data indicated that hopelessness, current quality of life, and fatigue were the most ardent predictors of feeling a burden to others. Of note, there was a lack of association between sense of burden to others and the actual degree of physical dependency, suggesting the perception of feeling burdensome is largely mediated through psychological and existential considerations.[20]

Aftermath Concerns

Unlike many of the other themes and subthemes contained within the Model of Dignity, Aftermath concerns are quite specific to patients facing end of life. These refer to the worries associated with anticipating the future burden or challenges that one's death will impose on others. While this type of psychological distress is similar to burden to others, it refers specifically to worries that the patient has about the impact death will have on those who are left behind. A 51-year-old outpatient with metastatic lung cancer expressed his aftermath concerns regarding the future of this children and how they would fare in the wake of his death. "Well I've got four children. They're all at home still. And my last boy, he's only age 12 and I'm really concerned about, you know, their future. Sometimes I worry about the family and things like that."[3] Dr Woelk recalled a palliative care patient he looked after recently, "a lady who was in her 40s. Her husband had had a brain injury, and was functioning fairly well, but she worried about him and what would become of him when she died. And she actually could tell me about those worries maybe more than she could tell her husband."

One young woman with end-stage lymphoma used Dignity Therapy as a way of trying to safeguard the well-being of people she would soon be leaving behind, especially her husband and their 18-month-old daughter. Her aftermath concerns revolved around the fact that her child would grow up without a mother and would likely have no memories of their time together. She also worried that sadness would engulf her husband, as well as her siblings and parents. In creating her legacy document, she addressed these concerns by telling her story, including the highlights of growing up, meeting her husband, their courtship and fairy-tale marriage. She devoted considerable attention to describing motherhood and the events and feelings surrounding her daughter's first 18 months. Besides using Dignity Therapy as a means of preserving memories, she also offered words of guidance, including asking them not to stay sad forever. In an act of grace, she expressed the hope—hence giving permission—for her husband to start a new family with a new partner who would love her daugher as her own.

Another young patient facing an uncertain prognosis used Dignity Therapy as a way of trying to inform and guide his wife and their three children in case he died. His story was a rags-to-riches tale in which he'd overcome tremendous adversity to eventually become a successful business owner and stable family man. He shared the highlights of his troubled youth, the struggle to turn his life around, and how he applied himself to his chosen trade. He told the story

of how he and his wife met, their marriage, and the transformative experience of becoming a father. In speaking about his children, he said his biggest
heartache was thinking about them growing up without him. In expressing
his wishes for his children, he emphasized the importance of education, physical activity, choosing a solid job, and avoiding some of the mistakes that he
had made along the way. He, too, hoped his family would overcome their grief
and that his wife would find a partner to share her life with. He assured his
family that, wherever he is, he would be watching over them.

References

1. Van Der Maas PJ, Van Delden JJ, Pijnenborg L, Looman CW. Euthanasia and other medical decisions concerning the end of life. Lancet. 1991;338:669–674.
2. Chochinov HM, Hack T, Hassard T, Kristjanson LJ, McClement S, Harlos M. Dignity in the terminally ill: A cross-sectional, cohort study. Lancet. 2002;360:2026–2030.
3. Chochinov HM, Hack T, McClement S, Harlos M, Kristjanson L. Dignity in the terminally ill: A developing empirical model. Soc Sci Med. 2002;54:433–443.
4. Chochinov HM, McClement SE, Hack TF, McKeen NA, Rach AM, Gagnon P, Sinclair S, Taylor-Brown J. The Patient Dignity Inventory: Applications in the oncology setting. J Palliat Med. 2012;15:998–1005.
5. Chochinov HM, Hassard T, McClement S, Hack T, Kristjanson LJ, Harlos M, Sinclair S, Murray A. The patient dignity inventory: A novel way of measuring dignity-related distress in palliative care. J Pain Symptom Manage. 2008;36:559–571.
6. Chochinov HM, Hack T, Hassard T, McClement S, Kristjanson L, Harlos M, Murray A, Sinclair S. The landscape of distress in the terminally ill. J Pain Sympt Manage. 2009;38:641–649.
7. Chochinov HM. *Dignity therapy: Final words for final days*. Oxford University Press; 2011.
8. Julião M, Oliveira F, Nunes B, Vaz Carneiro A, Barbosa A. Efficacy of dignity therapy on depression and anxiety in Portuguese terminally ill patients: A phase II randomized con- trolled trial. J Palliat Med. 2014;17:688–695.
9. Chochinov HM, Wilson K, Enns M, Lander S. Depression, hopelessness, and suicidal idea- tion in the terminally ill. Psychosomatics. 1998;39:366–370.
10. Chochinov HM, Kristjanson L, Hack T, Hassard T, McClement S, Harlos M. Dignity in the terminally ill: Revisited. J Palliat Med. 2006;9:666–672.
11. Kishi Y, Robinson RG, Kosier JT. Suicidal ideation among patients with acute life- threatening physical illness: Patients with stroke, traumatic brain injury, myocardial in- farction, and spinal cord injury. Psychosomatics. 2001;42:382–390.
12. Chochinov HM, Tataryn D, Wilson K, Ennis M, Lander S. Prognostic awareness and the terminally ill. Psychosomatics. 2000;41:500–504.
13. Breitbart W. On the inevitability of death. Palliat Support Care. 2017;15(3):276–278. doi:10.1017/S1478951517000372
14. Dixit J. The art of now: Six steps to living in the moment. 2008. https://www.psychologyto day.com/ca/articles/200811/the-art-now-six-steps-living-in-the-moment
15. Puchalski C, Ferrell B, Virani R, Otis-Green S, Baird P, Bull J, Chochinov H, Handzo G, Nelson-Becker H, Prince-Paul M, Pugliese K, Sulmasy D. Improving the quality of spiritual care as a dimension of palliative care: The report of the Consensus Conference. J Palliat Med. 2009;12:885–904.

16. Sulmasy DP. The varieties of human dignity: A logical and conceptual analysis. Med Health Care Philos. 2013;16:937–944.
17. Morgan DD, Marston C, Barnard E, Farrow C. Conserving dignity and facilitating adaptation to dependency with intimate hygiene for people with advanced disease: A qualitative study. Palliat Med. 2021;35:1366–1377.
18. Meyer M, Donnelly M, Weerakoon P. "They're taking the place of my hands": perspectives of people using personal care. Disability Society. 2007;22:595–608
19. Mugumbate JR, Chereni A. Editorial: Now, the theory of Ubuntu has its space in social work. Afr J Social Work. 2020;10(1).
20. Chochinov HM, Kristjanson L, Hack T, Hassard T, McClement S, Harlos M. Burden to others and the terminally ill. J Pain Symptom Manage. 2007;34:463–471.

Will I Lose My Dignity

Will I lose my dignity, will someone care? Will I wake tomorrow, from this nightmare?

—Jonathan Larson, from the musical *Rent* (1996)

Epilogue

Dr. Woelk occasionally mentors medical students who are doing some of their training in rural Manitoba. A few years ago, one such student "mentioned that she wanted to go and see a palliative care patient with me sometime, and I said, 'well, of course.' But you know how summers go, she was busy for a while and then I had some holidays for a while and then it turned out that it was her last day and I said, 'I'm going somewhere today. If you can get out of what you're doing, you can come with me.' And she was very keen."

So we get in the car and we go for a ride and the patient's home is almost an hour away, so we had a good chance to talk about the things that we talk about in medicine, and in palliative care, like pain management, nausea management, how to switch opioids, how to affect different receptors in the treatment of nausea. We went through all kinds of things, and she was a bright young medical student, who's now a bright young doctor. So then we got to this lady's house. She was in her late 40s or early 50s with an advanced gynaecological cancer. She'd had really good care from her family physician in her community and from the attending gyne-oncologists in the city where she'd gone for chemotherapy. But she had now been referred to the palliative care program because she was getting weaker and weaker.

We went into her home and we sat down in the living room. She had some older teenage kids that came into and out of the room while we were sitting there with her husband and a few others, her parents and couple of siblings, or maybe a friend. They wanted to hear what we had to say. It was the student's role to be there and observe; she wasn't talking, she was just listening. So we listened to the patient's story and how things had evolved for her, the symptoms she was having and how she was feeling. Towards the end of our discussion, the patient said to me, "Would you examine me, because nobody's come around for a while to examine me?" I said, "Sure, where would you like me to do that?" And she said, "Well, let's go into the bedroom." And so, very slowly and painstakingly we walked with her into the bedroom, and she lay down on the bed and got under the covers a little. And we lifted up her shirt and felt her tummy, and of course, she had some ascites, and she had palpable tumours. She didn't look well at all. She looked like someone who was going to die soon, and, when we were done, I told her what I could feel and what I thought. We helped her back to the living room, and we answered a few more questions. Then we said our goodbyes. We got back into the car, and I backed off of the driveway and started to drive, when I looked over and said, "So what do you think about all that, what just happened there?" She welled up with tears and she said, "I'm going to need to be a lot tougher if I'm going to do this kind of work."

Dignity in Care

This book has been written to describe the human side of healthcare, to help anyone doing this kind of work provide dignity in care, irrespective of disciplinary affiliation or clinical role. Dr. Woelk and his student found themselves engaging a patient and her family living in the grips of a healthcare crisis that threatened to change their lives forever. While his student opines that she needs to be *tougher*, dignity in care asserts that there is so much more to be considered.

This book began by having us consider the complexities of patienthood and the multitude of factors influencing patients' responses to changing health circumstances. In this instance, Dr. Woelk introduces us to his patient—a mother, a daughter, a wife, a friend—forced to adjust to living with advanced, metastatic gynecological cancer. Her transition into patienthood was no doubt shaped by the insidious nature of gynecological cancers, the uncertainies of this diagnosis, and the perceived bodily threat these spreading tumors impose. This process likely evolved with the emergence of each new symptom, each new piece of diagnostic information, and each new limitation or accommodation imposed by her disease.

While already well down the road into patienthood, one can imagine she remained engaged in relationships and community as a means of asserting personhood and not letting the physical and mental challenges of advanced cancer define her. Dr. Woelk's visit marked the beginning of a palliative care approach, suggesting she was about to enter a new phase of patienthood, one where comfort measures and quality of life would supercede prior efforts to offer cure or significant life extension. Being surrounded by family who were keen to hear Dr. Woelk's impressions suggests she was supported and loved and that her life still mattered to those with whom she was connected.

The ABCDs of Dignity Conserving Care, described in Chapter 2, highlight the importance of core competencies informing healthcare provider outlooks toward patients and their families and that are needed to achieve dignity in care. The essence of the ABCDs is that our disposition toward patients and families has a profound influence on their overall experience of healthcare.

Our Attitude, Behaviour, Compassion, and Dialogue that acknowledges personhood or elicits the *patient's thread* are critical ingredients of dignity in care. Dr. Woelk clearly felt that seeing this patient in her home was important, and he drove nearly an hour each way to do so, demonstrating caring and an investment in her well-being. In their first meeting, he was able to find out who this woman was and how she felt about what was happening to her. She clearly needed to tell her story, sharing the details of her anguish and concerns. Compassion demands that we understand the patient's subjective experience and perceived suffering, allowing for a virtues-based response meant to mitigate their underlying distress. This should also be informed by the Platinum Rule, which sees us consider treating patients not necessarily as *we* would want to be treated, but how *they* would want to be treated and cared for. Fulfilling her wish to be examined was an act of compassion, providing her information about her clinical status and reassurance that she still mattered.

The third chapter provides a unique way of understanding the anatomy of effective therapeutic communication, vital to achieving dignity in care. The Model of Optimal Therapeutic Effectiveness describes a detailed communication framework that enables the best possible clinical outcomes. This framework allows healthcare providers to identify elements required to optimize dignity in care within any given clinical encounter. The model specifies a number of key communication ingredients, including identifying a therapeutic task, ensuring that this task is delivered in a safe milieu, and that clinical encounters are informed and often transformed by healthcare practitioners introducing elements of the self. The model also highlights the importance of therapeutic pacing, therapeutic presence, and therapeutic humility.

The meeting with Dr. Woelk's patient can be examined through the lense of *optimal therapeutic communication*. The designated task was to meet the patient, introduce the notion of palliative care, and determine her specific needs and concerns. This was done with skill, grace, and finesse. In this case, attentiveness to a safe milieu was facilitated by way of seeing the patient in her own home. This was her space, her turf, which she shared with people who held her dear. One can only infer the elements of self, falling under the rubric of personal growth and self-care, that Dr. Woelk brought into this clinical encounter. He himself is a parent of young adult children and someone who has experienced the death of loved ones. In recounting this home visit, it is clear that whatever emotional reservoir he was tapping into, he was keenly aware of the pathos of this unfolding drama within which he had been called upon to be a key player.

Sensitive therapeutic pacing allowed this woman to reveal her story without a sense of being rushed, with questioning that was neither confrontative nor avoidant. Therapeutic presence—that is, Dr. Woelk being compassionate, nonjudgmental, genuine, trustworthy, and fully present—shaped this meeting into one that felt safe and nurturing. Elements of therapeutic humility also influenced the texture of this first meeting, in that the patient's agenda, wants, and needs were not entirely predictable. This means being comfortable with clinical ambiguity, not assuming that one has all the answers, and having faith in yielding to the clinical process.

The previous chapter, "Dignity in Care," details an empirical model offering healthcare providers a framework within which to understand various sources of dignity related distress. This model captures areas to keep on our clinical radar to preserve patient dignity. Being a competent and experienced palliative care physician, Dr. Woelk was attentive to his patient's illness-related concerns, identifying whatever symptom burden needed to be addressed to optimize her comfort. He was also prepared to answer questions to allay medical uncertainty, depending on her need for prognostic information and anticipation of her future disease course. But he was also interested in her story, including elements contained within the dignity-conserving repertoire. What is her thread? Can we locate personhood? What is her sense of continuity of self or role preservation? What does she still take pride in, and what gives her a sustained sense of hope, meaning, and purpose. What about her spiritual life? The request to be examined speaks to "Am I still worthy of your attention?" And performing an examination in the privacy of her bedroom was as much a diagnostic endeavor as it was a profound act of therapeutic affirmation.

For this patient, the Social Dignity Inventory reminds us that she is very much embedded in an extended family that care about her and that her fate and their well-being and emotional security are inextricably connected. Their presence is a constant reminder that she matters, that she is deserving of honor, respect, and esteem, which is the essence of dignity. Their image of her helps her sustain a sense of self-worth. The other element of the Social Dignity Inventory on prominent display during that visit was *care tenor*, or what was earlier referred to as the *fragrance of care*. These are ineffable qualities that Dr. Woelk embodies, which largely overlap with the construct of therapeutic presence within the Model of Optimal Therapeutic Effectiveness (see Chapter 3). Care tenor can be invoked independently of what one does to or with a patient or what one says. Rather, it is a way of *being* with a patient, a way that affirms their sense of dignity. When he asked his student, "So what do you think about all that, what just happened there?" dignity in care offers this textured response.

Dignity in care is relevant at the beginning of life, toward the end of life, and at all points in between. And dignity in care matters, not only to physicians and nurses, but to social workers, healthcare aides, hospital chaplains, occupational therapists, physiotherapists, physician's assistants, x-ray technologists, radiation therapists, respiratory therapists, pharmacists, medical receptionists, and triage nurses, among others, and healthcare trainees of all stripes. And, of course, dignity in care matters to healthcare consumers, whomever and wherever they happen to be. Those of us working in healthcare need to be mindful that patients are on a journey, most often not of their choosing. Understanding their struggle and the dynamics of how patienthood can overshadow personhood offers insight into how and why patients respond as they do. Being ever mindful of the ABCDs of dignity-conserving care ensures that healthcare providers are always aware that their presence, and the person they bring to the bedside, profoundly shapes each clinical encounter. The Model of Optimal Therapeutic Effectiveness unpacks elements of effective communication in a novel way, detailing those ingredients that need to be invoked if we are to achieve optimal therapeutic outcomes and dignity in care. Finally the Model of Dignity offers an empirical map that describes various issues and patient characteristics one must consider in providing dignity in care.

Changing health circumstances and disease can assault patients' sense of bodily integrity, disrupting function and comfort. All too often, when the human side of medicine is neglected, healthcare providers unwittingly inflict further harm, undermining patients' feelings of being understood and nurtured as they navigate their way through the healthcare system. The impact of this psychological and spiritual assault can be profound, fracturing identity and sense of personhood, eroding trust, and thus yielding poorer healthcare outcomes and diminished quality of life. Dignity in care is a way of preventing this iatrogenic injury, wherein the human side of medicine is embedded into the foundation of quality, compassionate healthcare. Patients and families deserve this kind of care. Healthcare providers deserve the rewards of engaging in patient connections that are truly healing, enhancing their satisfaction in caring and staving off the numbing disengagement that is a harbinger of professional burnout. All of us connected to healthcare, those who provide it and those who receive it, deserve a healthcare system that ascribes to dignity in care, one wherein *care* and *caring* are utterly indivisible. Dignity in care transforms healthcare into *healthcaring*. Anything less simply will not do.

And so this book ends as it started, and that is by having you look in the mirror. The reflection you see is someone whose contribution to patient care goes beyond the technical skillset and knowledge you bring. You are also a person with qualities and characteristics that will inform, shape, and transform each and every clinical encounter. So remember your ABCDs. Remember the tone or *fragrance* of care. Remember the Platinum Rule. And when all else fails and the overwhelming din of high-intensity, rapid-pace healthcare has you struggling to get a foothold in dignity in care, remember . . . *patients are people with feelings that matter.*

Index

For the benefit of digital users, indexed terms that span two pages (e.g., 52–53) may, on occasion, appear on only one of those pages.

Tables, figures, and boxes are indicated by *t*, *f*, and *b* following the page number